Look This Up, Too!
(A Quick Reference in Apheresis)
3rd Edition

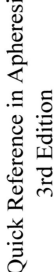

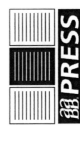

American Society for Apheresis

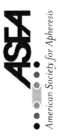

AABB PRESS

Other related publications from the AABB:

Look It Up! (A Quick Reference in Transfusion Medicine), 2nd edition
By Mark E. Brecher, MD, and Shauna Hay, MT(ASCP)

Therapeutic Apheresis: A Physician's Handbook, 4th edition
Edited by Jeffrey L. Winters, MD, and Karen King, MD

Apheresis: Principles and Practice, 3rd edition (book or CD-ROM)
Edited by Bruce C. McLeod, MD; Robert Weinstein, MD; Jeffrey L. Winters, MD; and Zbigniew M. Szczepiorkowski, MD, PhD, FCAP

The AABB Press produces hard copy and electronic publications on many topics of interest to those in the blood banking, transfusion medicine, and cellular therapy fields.

To purchase books or to inquire about other book services, including digital downloads and large-quantity sales, please contact our sales department:

- 866.222.2498 (within the United States)
- +1 301.215.6499 (outside the United States)
- +1 301.951.7150 (fax)
- www.aabb.org>Resources>Marketplace

AABB customer service representatives are available by telephone from 8:30 am to 5:00 pm ET, Monday through Friday, excluding holidays.

Look This Up, Too!
(A Quick Reference in Apheresis)
3rd Edition

Editors
Mark E. Brecher, MD
Beth H. Shaz, MD
Joseph (Yossi) Schwartz, MD

AABB Press
Bethesda, Maryland
2013

Mention of specific products or equipment by contributors to this AABB Press publication does not represent an endorsement of such products by the AABB Press nor does it necessarily indicate a preference for those products over other similar competitive products.

Efforts are made to have publications of the AABB Press consistent in regard to acceptable practices. However, for several reasons, they may not be. First, as new developments in the practice of blood banking occur, changes may be recommended to the AABB *Standards for Blood Banks and Transfusion Services*. It is not possible, however, to revise each publication at the time such a change is adopted. Thus, it is essential that the most recent edition of the *Standards* be consulted as a reference in regard to current acceptable practices. Second, the views expressed in this publication represent the opinions of authors. The publication of this book does not constitute an endorsement by the AABB Press of any view expressed herein, and the AABB Press expressly disclaims any liability arising from any inaccuracy or misstatement.

Copyright © 2013 by AABB. All rights reserved. Reproduction or transmission of text in any form or by any means, electronic or mechanical, including photocopying, recording, or by any information storage and retrieval system is prohibited without permission in writing from the Publisher.

The Publisher has made every effort to trace the copyright holders for borrowed material. If any such material has been inadvertently overlooked, the Publisher will be pleased to make the necessary arrangements at the first opportunity.

AABB
8101 Glenbrook Road
Bethesda, Maryland 20814-2749

ISBN NO. 978-1-56395-868-7
Printed in the United States

AABB Press
Editorial Board

Miguel Lozano, MD, PhD
Richard J. Davey, MD
Susan T. Johnson, MSTM, MT(ASCP)SBB
Marisa B. Marques, MD
Sally V. Rudmann, PhD, MT(ASCP)SBB
John W. Semple, PhD
Yan Yun Wu, MD, PhD

Table of Contents

Section 2. Calculations

Section 4. Donor Practice

Section 5. Cellular Therapy

Preface

Look This Up, Too! (A Quick Reference in Apheresis), now in its third edition, is updated with the publication of the new American Society for Apheresis Guidelines on the Use of Therapeutic Apheresis in Clinical Practice. In addition, new and revised tables are drawn principally from a variety of AABB publications (and a few selected other sources), while others have been created for this publication. The book gathers together an extensive collection of tables and figures that provide a succinct summary of information in apheresis medicine.

This publication is intended to provide a source of information that is frequently needed in the daily practice of therapeutic, donor, and cellular therapy apheresis. Use of apheresis textbooks and the American Society for Apheresis Guidelines will still need to be consulted for in-depth information.

Thanks to the AABB Press Editorial Board for recognizing the value of *Look This Up, Too!* and continuing to support its revisions, to AABB staff for helping with the publication, and to the American Society for Apheresis for its support.

Mark E. Brecher, MD
Chapel Hill, NC
Beth H. Shaz, MD
New York, NY
Joseph (Yossi) Schwartz, MD
New York, NY

xii

About the Editors

Mark E. Brecher, MD, is chief medical officer, interim chief scientific officer, and a senior vice president of the Laboratory Corporation of America. He is also an adjunct professor of pathology and laboratory medicine at the University of North Carolina at Chapel Hill. In 1982, Dr. Brecher received his BA (chemistry) from Emory University and his medical degree from the University of Chicago, where he also completed a surgical internship and a residency in anatomic/clinical pathology. He received fellowship training in blood bank/transfusion medicine at the Mayo Clinic and continued as a staff physician with the Mayo Clinic Blood Bank and Transfusion Service from 1988 through 1992. From 1992 through 2009 he was on the faculty at the University of North Carolina (Department of Pathology and Laboratory Medicine), most recently as professor and vice-chair for clinical services.

In addition to serving on the editorial boards of *TRANSFUSION* and *Journal of Clinical Apheresis*, Dr. Brecher is an ad hoc reviewer for many periodicals. He has published over 160 articles, commentaries, letters, and editorials, and 30 book chapters. He has edited 18 books, including during his time as chief editor of AABB's *Technical Manual* (14th and 15th editions) and *Collected Questions and Answers* (6th-10th editions).

Dr. Brecher is a member of several professional societies, including the AABB, College of American Pathologists (CAP), and American Society for Apheresis (ASFA). He has served on several AABB, CAP, American Society of Hematology (ASH), and ASFA committees. He is a past chair of the US Department of Health and Human Services Blood Safety and Availability Committee and a past president of ASFA.

Beth H. Shaz, MD, is chief medical officer, vice president of medical programs and services, transfusion medicine fellowship program director, and a member in the Lindsley F. Kimball Research Institute at New York Blood Center. She is a clinical associate professor at Emory University. Previously, Dr. Shaz was director of transfusion services at Grady Memorial Hospital in Atlanta, was an associate professor in the Department of Pathology and Laboratory Medicine at Emory University School of Medicine, and served as program director for the Emory Center of Transfusion and Cellular Therapies Transfusion Medicine Fellowship and the International Visiting Scholars Program. Previous to her service at Emory, she was an instructor at Harvard Medical School, assistant medical director of the transfusion service, and medical director of the transfusion/pheresis unit at Beth Israel Deaconess Medical Center. Nationally, she serves on the AABB Board of Directors and the Board of Trustees of National Blood Foundation, and is on the College of American Pathologists Transfusion Medicine Resource Committee.

Dr. Shaz has published over 60 peer-reviewed articles and 60 book chapters, is an associate editor of *TRANSFUSION*, and is on the editorial board of the *Journal of Clinical Apheresis*. She has coedited four books: *Transfusion Medicine and Hemostasis: Clinical Laboratory Aspects* (first and second editions) and *Look This Up, Too! (A Quick Reference in Apheresis)* (first and second editions).

Dr. Shaz graduated from Cornell University with distinction, majoring in chemical engineering, and from the University of Michigan Medical School with research distinction. She completed a surgical internship at Georgetown University, followed by pathology residency and transfusion medicine fellowship at Beth Israel Deaconess Medical Center, Harvard Medical School.

Joseph (Yossi) Schwartz, MD, is the director of the Transfusion Medicine and Cellular Therapy section at Columbia University Medical Center/New York Presbyterian Hospital (CUMC/NYPH). He is also an associate professor of Clinical Pathology and Cell Biology at Columbia University School of Medicine.

Dr. Schwartz received his medical degree from the Technion, Institute of Technology, Israel. He then completed an internal medicine residency, followed by a hematology fellowship. He had further training in blood bank/transfusion medicine in the Transfusion Medicine Fellowship Program of the New York Blood Center. He remained at the blood center as assistant medical director of the mobile apheresis service. He subsequently moved to CUMC/NYPH as the assistant medical director of the transfusion service and director of cell therapy and apheresis; currently, as the medical director of the Transfusion Medicine and Cellular Therapy section, he oversees the blood bank, apheresis, and cell therapy.

Dr. Schwartz has authored or coauthored approximately 80 articles, commentaries, letters, and editorials, and 10 book chapters in the areas of hematology, transfusion medicine, apheresis, and cell therapy. In addition to serving on the editorial board of the *Journal of Clinical Apheresis*, Dr. Schwartz is an ad hoc reviewer for many periodicals, including *TRANSFUSION*. Dr. Schwartz is a member of several professional societies, including the AABB, ASH, and ASFA. He serves on several AABB, ASFA, and CAP committees and currently serves on ASFA's Board of Directors. He is also the chair of the Standards Committee for the sixth edition of The Foundation for the Accreditation of Cellular Therapy–The Joint Accreditation Committee-ISCT (Europe) and EBMT (FACT–JACIE) standards.

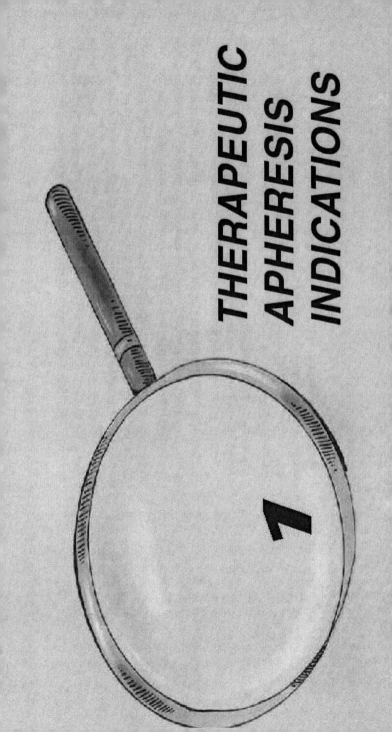

1

THERAPEUTIC APHERESIS INDICATIONS

Table 1-1. Apheresis Procedure Definitions*

Procedure/Term	Definition
Adsorptive cytapheresis	A therapeutic procedure in which blood of the patient is passed through a medical device which contains a column or filter that selectively adsorbs activated monocytes and granulocytes, allowing the remaining leukocytes and other blood components to be returned to the patient.
Apheresis	A procedure in which blood of the patient or donor is passed through a medical device which separates out one or more components of blood and returns the remainder with or without extracorporeal treatment or replacement of the separated component.
Erythrocytapheresis	A procedure in which blood of the patient or donor is passed through a medical device which separates red blood cells from other components of blood; the red blood cells are removed and replaced with crystalloid or colloid solution, when necessary.
Extracorporeal photopheresis (ECP)	A therapeutic procedure in which buffy coat, separated from the patient's blood, is treated extracorporeally with a photoactive compound (eg, psoralens) and exposed to ultraviolet A light and subsequently reinfused to the patient during the same procedure.
Filtration selective removal	A procedure which uses a filter to remove components from the blood based upon size. Depending upon the pore size of the filters used, different components can be removed. Filtration-based instruments can be used to perform plasma exchange or

LDL apheresis. They can also be used to perform donor plasmapheresis where plasma is collected for transfusion or further manufacture.

Immunoadsorption (IA)

A therapeutic procedure in which plasma of the patient, after separation from the blood, is passed through a medical device which has a capacity to remove immunoglobulins by specifically binding them to the active component (eg, Staphylococcal protein A) of the device.

LDL Apheresis

The selective removal of low-density lipoproteins from the blood, with the return of the remaining components. A variety of instruments are available which remove LDL cholesterol based upon charge (dextran sulfate and polyacrylate), size (double-membrane filtration), precipitation at low pH (HELP), or immunoadsorption with anti-Apo B-100 antibodies.

Leukocytapheresis (LCP)

A procedure in which blood of the patient or the donor is passed through a medical device which separates out white blood cells (eg, leukemic blasts or granulocytes), collects the selected cells, and returns the remainder of the patient's or the donor's blood with or without addition of replacement fluid such as colloid and/or crystalloid solution. This procedure can be used therapeutically or in preparation of blood components.

(cont'd)

Table 1-1. Apheresis Procedure Definitions* (Continued)

Procedure/Term	Definition
Plasma exchange (TPE)	A therapeutic procedure in which blood of the patient is passed through a medical device which separates out plasma from other components of blood; the plasma is removed and replaced with a replacement solution such as colloid solution (eg, albumin and/or plasma) or a combination of crystalloid/colloid solution.
Plasmapheresis	A procedure in which blood of the patient or the donor is passed through a medical device which separates out plasma from other components of blood, and the plasma is removed (ie, less than 15% of total plasma volume) without the use of replacement solution.
Plateletapheresis	A procedure in which blood of the donor is passed through a medical device which separates out platelets, collects the platelets, and returns the remainder of the donor's blood. This procedure is used in preparation of blood components (eg, apheresis platelets).
RBC exchange	A therapeutic procedure in which blood of the patient is passed through a medical device which separates red blood cells from other components of blood; the red blood cells are removed and replaced with donor red blood cells alone and colloid solution.

Rheopheresis	A therapeutic procedure in which blood of the patient is passed through a medical device which separates out high-molecular-weight plasma components such as fibrinogen, $\alpha2$-macroglobulin, LDL cholesterol, and IgM in order to reduce plasma viscosity and red cell aggregation. This is done to improve blood flow and tissue oxygenation. LDL apheresis devices and selective filtration devices utilizing two filters, one to separate plasma from cells and a second to separate the high-molecular-weight components, are used for these procedures.
Therapeutic apheresis (TA)	A therapeutic procedure in which blood of the patient is passed through an extracorporeal medical device which separates components of blood to treat a disease. This is a general term which includes all apheresis-based procedures used therapeutically.
Thrombocytapheresis	A therapeutic procedure in which blood of the patient is passed through a medical device which separates out platelets, removes the platelets, and returns the remainder of the patient's blood with or without addition of replacement fluid such as colloid and/or crystalloid solution.

*Modified from Schwartz J, Winters JL, Padmanabhan A, et al. Guidelines on the use of therapeutic apheresis in clinical practice—Evidence-based approach from the Apheresis Applications Committee of the American Society for Apheresis. The Sixth Special Issue. J Clin Apheresis 2013;28: 145-284.

Apo = apolipoprotein; HELP = heparin-induced extracorporeal LDL precipitation; LDL = low-density lipoprotein; TPE = therapeutic plasma exchange.

Table 1-2. Indications for Therapeutic Apheresis—ASFA 2013 Categories*

Category	Description
I	Disorders for which apheresis is accepted as first-line therapy, either as a primary stand-alone treatment or in conjunction with other modes of treatment. [Example: plasma exchange in Guillain-Barré syndrome as first-line standalone therapy; plasma exchange in myasthenia gravis as first-line therapy in conjunction with immunosuppression and cholinesterase inhibition].
II	Disorders for which apheresis is accepted as second-line therapy, either as a standalone treatment or in conjunction with other modes of treatment. [Example: plasma exchange as stand-alone secondary treatment for acute disseminated encephalomyelitis after high-dose IV corticosteroid failure; extracorporeal photopheresis added to corticosteroids for unresponsive chronic graft-versus-host disease]
III	Optimum role of apheresis therapy is not established. Decision making should be individualized. [Example: extracorporeal photopheresis for nephrogenic systemic fibrosis; plasma exchange in patients with sepsis and multiorgan failure]

IV   Disorders in which published evidence demonstrates or suggests apheresis to be ineffective or harmful. IRB approval is desirable if apheresis treatment is undertaken in these circumstances. [Example: plasma exchange for active rheumatoid arthritis]

*Modified from Schwartz J, Winters JL, Padmanabhan A, et al. Guidelines on the use of therapeutic apheresis in clinical practice—Evidence-based approach from the Apheresis Applications Committee of the American Society for Apheresis. The Sixth Special Issue. J Clin Apheresis 2013;28: 145-284.

ASFA = American Society for Apheresis; IRB = institutional review board; IV = intravenous.

Table 1-3. Grading Recommendations*

Recommendation	Description	Methodological Quality of Supporting Evidence	Implications
Grade 1A	Strong recommendation, high-quality evidence	RCTs without important limitations or overwhelming evidence from observational studies	Strong recommendation, can apply to most patients in most circumstances without reservation
Grade 1B	Strong recommendation, moderate quality evidence	RCTs with important limitations (inconsistent results, methodological flaws, indirect, or imprecise) or exceptionally strong evidence from observational studies	Strong recommendation, can apply to most patients in most circumstances without reservation
Grade 1C	Strong recommendation, low-quality or very low-quality evidence	Observational studies or case series	Strong recommendation but may change when higher-quality evidence becomes available

Grade 2A	Weak recommendation, high-quality evidence	RCTs without important limitations or overwhelming evidence from observational studies	Weak recommendation, best action may differ depending on circumstances or patients' or societal values
Grade 2B	Weak recommendation, moderate-quality evidence	RCTs with important limitations (inconsistent results, methodological flaws, indirect, or imprecise) or exceptionally strong evidence from observational studies	Weak recommendation, best action may differ depending on circumstances or patients' or societal values
Grade 2C	Weak recommendation, low-quality or very low-quality evidence	Observational studies or case series	Very weak recommendations; other alternatives may be equally reasonable

*Modified from Schwartz J, Winters JL, Padmanabhan A, et al. Guidelines on the use of therapeutic apheresis in clinical practice—Evidence-based approach from the Apheresis Applications Committee of the American Society for Apheresis. The Sixth Special Issue. J Clin Apheresis 2013;28:145-284.

RCT = randomized controlled trial.

Table 1-4. Modified McLeod's Criteria for Evaluation of Efficacy of Therapeutic Apheresis*

Evidence	McLeod's Criteria	Explanation
Mechanism	"Plausible Pathogenesis"	The current understanding of the disease process supports a clear rationale for the use of therapeutic apheresis modality.
Correction	"Better Blood"	The abnormality, which makes therapeutic apheresis plausible, can be meaningfully corrected by its use.
Clinical Effect	"Perkier Patients"	There is a strong evidence that therapeutic apheresis confers benefit that is clinically worthwhile, and not just statistically significant

*Modified from Schwartz J, Winters JL, Padmanabhan A, et al. Guidelines on the use of therapeutic apheresis in clinical practice—Evidence-based approach from the Apheresis Applications Committee of the American Society for Apheresis. The Sixth Special Issue. J Clin Apheresis 2013;28:145-284.

Table 1-5. ASFA 2013 Indication Categories for Therapeutic Apheresis*

Disease Name	Special Condition	Therapeutic Apheresis Modality	Category	Recommendation Grade
Acute disseminated encephalomyelitis		TPE	II	2C
Acute inflammatory demyelinating polyneuropathy (Guillain-Barré syndrome)		TPE	I	1A
	Post IVIG	TPE	III	2C
Acute liver failure		TPE	III	2B
Age-related macular degeneration, dry		Rheopheresis	I	1B
Amyloidosis, systemic		TPE	IV	2C
Amyotrophic lateral sclerosis		TPE	IV	1C

(cont'd)

11

Table 1-5. ASFA 2013 Indication Categories for Therapeutic Apheresis* (Continued)

Disease Name	Special Condition	Therapeutic Apheresis Modality	Category	Recommendation Grade
ANCA-associated rapidly progressive glomerulone-phritis (granulomatosis with polyangiitis; Wegener granulomatosis)	Dialysis dependence	TPE	I	1A
	DAH	TPE	I	1C
	Dialysis independence	TPE	III	2C
Antiglomerular basement membrane disease (Goodpasture syndrome)	Dialysis dependence and no DAH	TPE	III	2B
	DAH	TPE	I	1C
	Dialysis independence	TPE	I	1B
Aplastic anemia; pure red cell aplasia	Aplastic anemia	TPE	III	2C
	Pure red cell aplasia	TPE	III	2C

12

Autoimmune hemolytic anemia—warm autoimmune hemolytic anemia; cold agglutinin disease			
	Severe warm autoimmune hemolytic anemia	TPE	III	2C
	Severe cold agglutinin disease	TPE	II	2C
Babesiosis	Severe	RBC exchange	I	1C
	High-risk population	RBC exchange	II	2C
Burn shock resuscitation		TPE	III	2B
Cardiac transplantation	Rejection prophylaxis	ECP	II	2A
	Cellular or recurrent rejection	ECP	II	1B
	Desensitization, positive cross-match due to donor-specific HLA antibody	TPE	III	2C
	Antibody-mediated rejection	TPE	III	2C
Catastrophic antiphospholipid syndrome		TPE	II	2C

(cont'd)

13

Table 1-5. ASFA 2013 Indication Categories for Therapeutic Apheresis* (Continued)

Disease Name	Special Condition	Therapeutic Apheresis Modality	Category	Recommendation Grade
Chronic focal encephalitis (Rasmussen encephalitis)		TPE	III	2C
		IA	III	2C
Chronic inflammatory demyelinating polyradiculoneuropathy		TPE	I	1B
Coagulation factor inhibitors	Alloantibody	TPE	IV	2C
	Alloantibody	IA	III	2B
	Autoantibody	TPE	III	2C
	Autoantibody	IA	III	1C
Cryoglobulinemia	Symptomatic/severe	TPE	I	2A
	Symptomatic/severe	IA	II	2B

14

Disease	Subgroup	Treatment	Category	Grade
Cutaneous T-cell lymphoma—mycosis fungoides; Sézary syndrome	Erythrodermic	ECP	I	1B
	Nonerythrodermic	ECP	III	2C
Dermatomyositis or polymyositis		TPE	IV	2A
		Leukocytapheresis	IV	2A
Dilated cardiomyopathy, idiopathic	NYHA II-IV	TPE	III	2C
	NYHA II-IV	IA	II	1B
Familial hypercholesterolemia	Homozygotes	LDL apheresis	I	1A
	Heterozygotes	LDL apheresis	II	1A
	Homozygotes with small blood volume	TPE	II	1C
Focal segmental glomerulosclerosis	Recurrent in transplanted kidney	TPE	I	1B

(cont'd)

15

Table 1-5. ASFA 2013 Indication Categories for Therapeutic Apheresis* (Continued)

Disease Name	Special Condition	Therapeutic Apheresis Modality	Category	Recommendation Grade
Graft-vs-host disease	Skin (chronic)	ECP	II	1B
	Skin (acute)	ECP	II	1C
	Non-skin (acute/chronic)	ECP	III	2B
Hematopoietic stem cell transplantation, ABO-incompatible	Major HPC, Marrow	TPE	II	1B
	Major HPC, Apheresis	TPE	II	2B
	Minor HPC, Apheresis	RBC exchange	III	2C
Hemolytic uremic syndrome, atypical	Complement gene mutations	TPE	II	2C
	Factor H antibodies	TPE	I	2C
	MCP mutations	TPE	IV	1C
Hemolytic uremic syndrome, infection-associated	Shiga toxin-associated	TPE	IV	1C
	Streptococcus pneumoniae-associated	TPE	III	2C

16

Henoch-Schonlein purpura	Crescentic	TPE	III	2C
	Severe extrarenal disease	TPE	III	2C
Heparin-induced thrombocyto-penia	Precardiopulmonary bypass	TPE	III	2C
	Thrombosis	TPE	III	2C
Hereditary hemochromatosis		Erythrocytapheresis	I	1B
Hyperleukocytosis	Leukostasis	Leukocytapheresis	I	1B
	Prophylaxis	Leukocytapheresis	III	2C
Hypertriglyceridemic pancre-atitis		TPE	III	2C
Hyperviscosity in monoclonal gammopathies	Symptomatic	TPE	I	1B
	Prophylaxis for rituximab	TPE	I	1C
Immune complex rapidly pro-gressive glomerulonephritis		TPE	III	2B

(cont'd)

17

Table 1-5. ASFA 2013 Indication Categories for Therapeutic Apheresis* (Continued)

Disease Name	Special Condition	Therapeutic Apheresis Modality	Category	Recommendation Grade
Immune thrombocytopenia	Refractory	TPE	IV	2C
	Refractory	IA	III	2C
Immunoglobin A nephropathy	Crescentic	TPE	III	2B
	Chronic progressive	TPE	III	2C
Inclusion body myositis		TPE	IV	2C
		Leukocytapheresis	IV	2C
Inflammatory bowel disease	Ulcerative colitis	Adsorptive cytapheresis	III/II	1B/2B
	Crohn disease	Adsorptive cytapheresis	III	1B
	Crohn disease	ECP	III	2C
Lambert-Eaton myasthenic syndrome		TPE	II	2C
Lipoprotein (a) hyperlipoproteinemia		LDL apheresis	II	1B

18

Liver transplantation, ABO-incompatible	Desensitization, live donor	TPE	I	1C
	Desensitization, deceased donor	TPE	III	2C
	Humoral rejection	TPE	III	2C
Lung allograft rejection	Bronchiolitis obliterans syndrome	ECP	II	1C
	Antibody-mediated rejection	TPE	III	2C
Malaria	Severe	RBC exchange	II	2B
Multiple sclerosis	Acute CNS inflammatory demyelinating disease	TPE	II	1B
	Acute CNS inflammatory demyelinating disease	IA	III	2C
	Chronic progressive	TPE	III	2B
Myasthenia gravis	Moderate-severe	TPE	I	1B
	Prethymectomy	TPE	I	1C

(cont'd)

19

Table 1-5. ASFA 2013 Indication Categories for Therapeutic Apheresis* (Continued)

Disease Name	Special Condition	Therapeutic Apheresis Modality	Category	Recommendation Grade
Myeloma cast nephropathy		TPE	II	2B
Nephrogenic sytemic fibrosis		ECP	III	2C
		TPE	III	2C
Neuromyelitis optica (Devic syndrome)	Acute	TPE	II	1B
	Maintenance	TPE	III	2C
Overdose, envenomation, and poisoning	Mushroom poisoning	TPE	II	2C
	Envenomation	TPE	III	2C
	Natalizumab and progressive multifocal leukoencephalopathy	TPE	III	2C
	Tacrolimus	RBC exchange	III	2C
Paraneoplastic neurologic syndromes		TPE	III	2C
		IA	III	2C

20

Disease	Condition	Treatment		
Paraproteinemic demyelinating polyneuropathies	IgG/IgA	TPE	I	1B
	IgM	TPE	I	1C
	Multiple myeloma	TPE	III	2C
	IgG/IgA/IgM	IA	III	2C
Pediatric autoimmune neuropsychiatric disorders associated with streptococcal infections (PANDAS) and Sydenham chorea	PANDAS (exacerbation)	TPE	I	1B
	Sydenham chorea	TPE	I	1B
Pemphigus vulgaris	Severe	TPE	III	2C
	Severe	ECP	III	2C
	Severe	IA	III	2C
Peripheral vascular diseases		LDL apheresis	III	2C
Phytanic acid storage disease (Refsum disease)		TPE	II	2C
		LDL apheresis	II	2C

21

(cont'd)

Table 1-5. ASFA 2013 Indication Categories for Therapeutic Apheresis* (Continued)

Disease Name	Special Condition	Therapeutic Apheresis Modality	Category	Recommendation Grade
Polycythemia vera and erythrocytosis	Polycythemia vera	Erythrocytapheresis	I	1B
	Secondary erythrocytosis	Erythrocytapheresis	III	1C
Polyneuropathy, organomegaly, endocrinopathy, M protein, and skin changes (POEMS)		TPE	IV	1C
Posttransfusion purpura		TPE	III	2C
Psoriasis		TPE	IV	2C
	Disseminated pustular	Adsorptive cytapheresis	III	2C
		Lymphocytapheresis	III	2C
		ECP	III	2B
Red cell alloimmunization in pregnancy	Before IUT availability	TPE	III	2C

22

Renal transplantation, ABO-compatible	Antibody-mediated rejection	TPE	I	1B
	Desensitization, living donor, positive crossmatch due to donor-specific HLA antibody	TPE	I	1B
	Desensitization, high PRA, deceased donor	TPE	III	2C
Renal transplantation, ABO-incompatible	Desensitization, live donor	TPE	I	1B
	Humoral rejection	TPE	II	1B
	Group A2/A2B into B, deceased donor	TPE	IV	1B
Schizophrenia		TPE	IV	1A
Scleroderma (progressive systemic sclerosis)		TPE	III	2C
		ECP	III	2B
Sepsis with multiorgan failure		TPE	III	2B

(cont'd)

23

Table 1-5. ASFA 2013 Indication Categories for Therapeutic Apheresis* (Continued)

Disease Name	Special Condition	Therapeutic Apheresis Modality	Category	Recommendation Grade
Sickle cell disease, acute	Acute stroke	RBC exchange	I	1C
	Acute chest syndrome, severe	RBC exchange	II	1C
	Priapism	RBC exchange	III	2C
	Multiorgan failure	RBC exchange	III	2C
	Splenic sequestration; hepatic sequestration; intrahepatic cholestasis	RBC exchange	III	2C
Sickle cell disease, nonacute	Stroke prophylaxis or iron overload prevention	RBC exchange	II	1C
	Vaso-occlusive pain crisis	RBC exchange	III	2C
	Preoperative management	RBC exchange	III	2A
Stiff-person syndrome		TPE	III	2C

Sudden sensorineural hearing loss		LDL apheresis	III	2A
		Rheopheresis	III	2A
		TPE	III	2C
Systemic lupus erythematosus	Severe	TPE	II	2C
	Nephritis	TPE	IV	1B
Thrombocytosis	Symptomatic	Thrombocytapheresis	II	2C
	Prophylactic or secondary	Thrombocytapheresis	III	2C
Thrombotic microangiopathy, drug-associated	Ticlopidine	TPE	I	1B
	Clopidogrel	TPE	III	2B
	Cyclosporine/ Tacrolimus	TPE	III	2C
	Gencitabine	TPE	IV	2C
	Quinine	TPE	IV	2C
Thrombotic microangiopathy, hematopoietic stem cell transplant-associated	Refractory	TPE	III	2C

(cont'd)

Table 1-5. ASFA 2013 Indication Categories for Therapeutic Apheresis* (Continued)

Disease Name	Special Condition	Therapeutic Apheresis Modality	Category	Recommendation Grade
Thrombotic thrombocytopenic purpura		TPE	I	1A
Thyroid storm		TPE	III	2C
Toxic epidermal necrolysis	Refractory	TPE	III	2B
Voltage-gated potassium channel antibodies		TPE	II	1C
Wilson disease	Fulminant	TPE	I	1C

*Modified from Schwartz J, Winters JL, Padmanabhan A, et al. Guidelines on the use of therapeutic apheresis in clinical practice—Evidence-based approach from the Apheresis Applications Committee of the American Society for Apheresis. The Sixth Special Issue. J Clin Apheresis 2013;28:145-284.

ANCA = antineutrophil cytoplasmic antibody; CNS = central nervous system; DAH = diffuse alveolar hemorrhage; ECP = extracorporeal photochemotherapy; HPC = hematopoietic progenitor cell; IA = immunoadsorption; Ig = immunoglobulin; IUT = intrauterine transfusion; IV = intravenous; LCP = leukocytapheresis; MCP = membrane cofactor protein; NA = not applicable; NYHA = New York Heart Association; PML = progressive multifocal leukoencephalopathy; PRA = panel-reactive antibody; RBC = red blood cell; TPE = therapeutic plasma exchange.

Table 1-6. Descriptions of Diseases for Which Therapeutic Apheresis Is Recommended*

ACUTE DISSEMINATED ENCEPHALOMYELITIS (ADEM)

Procedure	Recommendation	Category
TPE	Grade 2C	II
Volume treated: 1-1.5 TPV	**Frequency:** every other day	
Replacement fluid: albumin		

There is no clear standard from which to make recommendations as to the optimum use of TPE in ADEM. In the largest case study, TPE achieved moderate and marked sustained improvement in 50% of the patients. Factors associated with improvement were male sex, preserved reflexes, and early initiation of treatment. In most published literature, response was noticeable within days, usually after two to three exchanges. If improvement is not observed early in treatment, then it is unlikely a response will occur. TPE therapy consists of three to six treatments, most commonly five.

(cont'd)

Table 1-6. Descriptions of Diseases for Which Therapeutic Apheresis Is Recommended* (Continued)

ACUTE INFLAMMATORY DEMYELINATING POLYNEUROPATHY (AIDP; GUILLAIN-BARRÉ SYNDROME)

Condition	Procedure	Recommendation	Category
	TPE	Grade 1A	I
After IVIG	TPE	Grade 2C	III

Volume treated: 1-1.5 TPV   **Frequency:** every other day

Replacement fluid: albumin

The typical TPE strategy is to exchange 200 to 250 mL plasma per kg body weight over 10 to 14 days. This will generally require five to six TPE procedures with 5% albumin replacement. Plasma is not routinely used for replacement. Because autonomic dysfunction may be present, affected patients may be more susceptible to volume shifts and to blood pressure and heart rate changes during extracorporeal treatment. Relapses may occur in approximately 10% of patients 2 to 3 weeks following either treatment with TPE or IVIG. When relapses occur, additional therapy, usually TPE, can be helpful. In AIDP patients with axonal involvement, TPE has been reported to be of greater potential benefit than IVIG. Frequently, when patients do not respond to IVIG, TPE is requested as the secondary therapy. Retrospective studies showed that such an approach has limited therapeutic benefit, yet it is significantly more expensive. Requests for TPE after IVIG treatment should be considered only in the context of each patient's clinical situation. Five to six TPEs over 10 to 14 days are recommended.

ACUTE LIVER FAILURE

Procedure	Recommendation	Category
TPE	Grade 2B	III

Volume treated: 1-1.5 TPV   **Frequency:** daily

Replacement fluid: plasma, albumin

Because plasma has citrate as an anticoagulant and there is significant hepatic dysfunction, the whole blood:ACD-A ratio should be adjusted accordingly to prevent severe hypocalcemia in acute liver failure. Simultaneous calcium infusion can be used if necessary. Patients should also be monitored for development of metabolic alkalosis. Some groups have performed simultaneous hemodialysis to mitigate this adverse event. There is a preference for plasma as a replacement fluid because of moderate to severe coagulopathy; however, addition of albumin is acceptable. Calcium supplementation should be strongly considered.

In acute liver failure, daily TPE is performed until transplantation or self-regeneration occurs. The biochemical response to TPE should be evaluated in laboratory values drawn the following day (≥12 hours or more after TPE). Samples drawn immediately after completion of the exchange would be expected to appear better compared to preexchange levels. Rarely TPE can be performed 2 to 3 times per week for 4 weeks in primary biliary cirrhosis to alleviate pruritus until a clinical response is observed.

(cont'd)

Table 1-6. Descriptions of Diseases for Which Therapeutic Apheresis Is Recommended* (Continued)

AGE RELATED MACULAR DEGENERATION, DRY (AMD)

Procedure	Recommendation	Category
Rheopheresis	Grade 1B	I
Volume treated: 0.8-1.2 TPV	**Frequency:** 8-10 treatments (2 per week) over 8-21 weeks	
Replacement fluid: NA		

The majority of series and trials used double-filtration plasmapheresis (DFPP). In this, plasma is separated by filtration and then passed through a second filter. Low-molecular-weight substances such as albumin pass through the filter, while high-molecular-weight substances are removed. These devices are not available in the United States. One case series did indicate that TPE with albumin replacement was used to treat AMD, but the trial included the use of other treatment modalities (eg, tryptophan polyvinyl alcohol columns and DFPP), and the authors provide inadequate information to determine whether there was a benefit with TPE.

Studies have suggested that those with elevations in high-molecular-weight plasma components have a better response, and that patients with dry AMD respond better than those with wet AMD. Efficacy of a single course has been reported to last for up to 4 years. One case series has suggested that after 12 months, two to four booster treatments could be considered, depending upon the patient's course.

Currently, the devices necessary for this treatment are not licensed in the United States but are available in Europe and Canada.

ANCA-ASSOCIATED RAPIDLY PROGRESSIVE GLOMERULONEPHRITIS (RPGN; GRANULOMATOSIS WITH POLYANGIITIS; WEGENER GRANULOMATOSIS)

Condition	Procedure	Recommendation	Category
Dialysis dependence*	TPE	Grade 1A	I
DAH	TPE	Grade 1C	I
Dialysis independence*	TPE	Grade 2C	III

Volume treated: 1-1.5 TPV   **Frequency:** daily or every other day

Replacement fluid: albumin; plasma when DAH present

*At presentation, defined as Cr >6 mg/dL.

Randomized controlled trials of TPE in patients with RPGN and pulmonary hemorrhage have not been conducted. However, a retrospective case series reported effective management of pulmonary hemorrhage in ANCA vasculitis.

Consider daily procedures in fulminant cases or with pulmonary hemorrhage, then continuing every 2 to 3 days for a total of six to nine procedures.

(cont'd)

31

Table 1-6. Descriptions of Diseases for Which Therapeutic Apheresis Is Recommended* (Continued)

ANTIGLOMERULAR BASEMENT MEMBRANE DISEASE (ANTI-GBM; GOODPASTURE SYNDROME)

Condition	Procedure	Recommendation	Category
Dialysis dependence*	TPE	Grade 2B	III
No DAH	TPE	Grade 1C	I
DAH	TPE	Grade 1B	I
Dialysis independence*			

Volume treated: 1-1.5 TPV **Frequency:** daily or every other day
Replacement fluid: albumin; plasma when DAH present

*At presentation, defined as Cr >6 mg/dL.

In most patients undergoing TPE and immunosuppression, GBM antibodies fall to undetectable levels within 2 weeks; thus, the minimum course of TPE should be 14 days. The presence or absence of antibody itself should not be used to initiate or terminate therapy, because antibody is not demonstrable in a few patients with the disease and may be present in patients without active disease. In patients with active disease, TPE should continue until resolution of evidence of ongoing glomerular or pulmonary injury. Of note, some studies have found that patients with DAH but no renal involvement do well regardless of the use of TPE.

APLASTIC ANEMIA; ACQUIRED PURE RED CELL APLASIA (PRCA)

Condition	Procedure	Recommendation	Category
Aplastic Anemia	TPE	Grade 2C	III
PRCA	TPE	Grade 2C	III

Volume treated: 1-1.5 TPV **Frequency:** daily or every other day

Replacement fluid: albumin, plasma

TPE is performed until recovery of hematopoiesis or adequate RBC production. No well-defined treatment schedules exist, although one to 24 treatments have been reported in the literature.

(cont'd)

Table 1-6. Descriptions of Diseases for Which Therapeutic Apheresis Is Recommended* (Continued)

AUTOIMMUNE HEMOLYTIC ANEMIA: WARM AUTOIMMUNE HEMOLYTIC ANEMIA (WAIHA); COLD AGGLUTININ DISEASE (CAD)

Condition	Procedure	Recommendation	Category
Severe WAIHA	TPE	Grade 2C	III
Severe CAD	TPE	Grade 2C	II

Volume treated: 1-1.5 TPV   **Frequency:** daily or every other day
Replacement fluid: albumin

If the thermal amplitude of an IgM cold autoantibody is such that agglutination occurs at room temperature, red cell agglutination may occur within the cell separator and tubing. In these situations, therapy may require a controlled, high temperature setting of 37 C both in the room and within the extracorporeal circuit.

TPE should be performed until hemolysis decreases and the need for transfusions is limited, or until drug therapy takes effect.

BABESIOSIS

Condition	Procedure	Recommendation	Category
Severe	RBC exchange	Grade 1C	I
High-risk population	RBC exchange	Grade 2C	II

Volume treated: 1-2 total RBC volume

Frequency: single procedure, but can be repeated

Replacement fluid: leukocyte-reduced RBCs

Automated apheresis instruments calculate the amount of red cells required to achieve the desired postprocedure Hct, fraction of red cells remaining and, by inference, the estimated final parasite load. A single two-volume RBC exchange can reduce the fraction of remaining patient red cells to roughly 10% to 15% of the original. In critically ill patients for whom antimicrobials and/or RBC exchange failed, the use of TPE has also been reported. For patients with severe coagulopathy, plasma may be incorporated into replacement fluid, either by performing whole blood exchange or TPE.

The specific threshold level of parasitemia for performing RBC exchange is not clear, but 10% is the most commonly used guideline, as well as severe symptoms. The specific level to which parasitemia must be reduced to elicit the maximum therapeutic effect is not clear, either. Treatment is usually discontinued after achieving <5% residual parasitemia. The decision to repeat the exchange is based on the level of parasitemia after exchange, as well as the clinical condition (ongoing signs and symptoms).

(cont'd)

35

Table 1-6. Descriptions of Diseases for Which Therapeutic Apheresis Is Recommended* (Continued)

BURN SHOCK RESUSCITATION

Procedure	Recommendation	Category
TPE	Grade 2B	III
Volume treated: 1.5 TPV	**Frequency:** once	
Replacement fluid: plasma, albumin		

TPE was instituted early in the postburn period, typically 8 to 16 hours after injury. Patients treated with TPE had greater than 20% to 50% total body surface area (TBSA) burns and were refractory to fluid resuscitation in most reports. In the retrospective historic controlled trial, TPE was initiated if the total resuscitation volumes exceeded 1.2 times the volume predicted by the modified Baxter formula (3 cm^3 LR/Kg/%TBSA) as necessary to keep urine output (UOP) >50 cm^3/hour and/or mean arterial pressure (MAP) ≥65 mm Hg. TPE adverse reactions were infrequently reported in these studies, although it is not clear if this was related to absence of adverse-reaction reporting in the case-study design or true tolerance of the TPE procedure.

In most reports, a TPE was performed within the first 24 hours (8-16 hours) after the burn, with an additional one or two TPE procedures in select patients. In the retrospective historic controlled trial, patients whose MAP and UOP did not increase or whose IV fluid volumes did not decline to predicted volumes received a second TPE within 6 to 8 hours of the first.

CARDIAC TRANSPLANTATION (HUMORAL/CELLULAR REJECTION; ABO COMPATIBLE)

Condition	Procedure	Recommendation	Category
Rejection prophylaxis	ECP	Grade 2A	II
Cellular/recurrent rejection	ECP	Grade 1B	II
Desensitization	TPE	Grade 2C	III
Antibody-mediated rejection	TPE	Grade 2C	III

Volume treated—ECP: MNC product is typically obtained after processing 1.5 L of blood (CELLEX/UVAR XTS); the two-step process method collects and treats MNCs obtained from two-TBV processing; **TPE:** 1-1.5 TPV

Frequency—ECP: two procedures on consecutive days (one series) weekly or every 2-8 weeks for several months (regimens vary widely); **TPE:** daily or every other day

Replacement fluid—ECP: NA; **TPE:** albumin, plasma

In low-body-weight patients, ECP may require protocol adjustments to compensate for the extracorporeal volume during the procedure. Although it is unknown whether a certain minimum dose of MNCs must be treated to mediate the benefits of ECP, it is advisable to draw a complete blood count before the procedure to ensure that there are circulating MNCs. Lymphopenia is not uncommon in this patient population.

There are no clear criteria for discontinuing treatment in ECP. Treatments are typically continued until improvement or stabilization of symptoms occurs. For TPE, improvement in cardiac function, biopsy findings, and donor-specific antibody levels are often used to determine timing of discontinuation of treatments.

(cont'd)

Table 1-6. Descriptions of Diseases for Which Therapeutic Apheresis Is Recommended* (Continued)

CATASTROPHIC ANTIPHOSPHOLIPID SYNDROME

Procedure	Recommendation	Category
TPE	Grade 2C	II

Volume treated: 1-1.5 TPV   **Frequency:** daily

Replacement fluid: plasma (albumin alone is rarely used)

Plasma was used in most reported cases; the efficacy of albumin has not been widely tested. Most published cases have reported daily TPE for a minimum of 3 to 5 days. Clinical response dictates the duration of TPE; no single clinical or laboratory parameter is used to determine when to discontinue treatment. Some patients have been treated for weeks instead of days.

38

CHRONIC FOCAL ENCEPHALITIS (RASMUSSEN ENCEPHALITIS)

Procedure	Recommendation	Category
TPE	Grade 2C	III
IA	Grade 2C	III

Volume treated—TPE: 1-1.5 TPV; **IA:** 1.5-2 TPV

Replacement fluid—TPE: albumin; **IA:** NA

Frequency—TPE: 3-6 TPEs over 6-12 days, repeated monthly; alternative schedule: TPE weekly; **IA:** 1-3, repeated monthly

Neuropsychological assessment may be helpful in evaluating patients with slowly progressive disease to determine whether TPE is effective in postponing surgical therapy. Protein A column treatment has not been directly compared to TPE. An initial course of TPE may be followed by 2 days of IVIG, 1 g/kg. A similar approach may be taken in subsequent courses if a salutary clinical effect is apparent. **Note:** Since December 2006, devices used to perform protein A immunoadsorption apheresis have not been commercially available in the United States.

After an initial course of treatment, subsequent courses of TPE (with or without IVIG) may be performed at intervals of 1 to 2 weeks or up to 2 to 3 months, as empirically needed to maintain clinical stability and avoid or delay hemispherectomy. Immunosuppressive medications may increase the interval between courses. Surgical treatment is offered for the management of patients who exhibit functional or cognitive decline or intractable seizure activity despite intensive immunomodulatory therapy.

(cont'd)

39

Table 1-6. Descriptions of Diseases for Which Therapeutic Apheresis Is Recommended* (Continued)

CHRONIC INFLAMMATORY DEMYELINATING POLYRADICULONEUROPATHY

Procedure	Recommendation	Category
TPE	Grade 1B	I
Volume treated: 1-1.5 TPV	**Frequency:** 2-3/week until improvement, then taper as tolerated	
Replacement fluid: albumin		

TPE provides short-term benefit, but rapid deterioration may occur afterwards. This may necessitate maintenance treatment, with TPE and/or other immunomodulating therapies, which should be tailored to the individual patient. The frequency of maintenance TPE may range from weekly to monthly, as needed to control symptoms.

COAGULATION FACTOR INHIBITORS

Condition	Procedure	Recommendation	Category
Alloantibody	TPE	Grade 2C	IV
Alloantibody	IA	Grade 2B	III
Autoantibody	TPE	Grade 2C	III
Autoantibody	IA	Grade 1C	III

Volume treated—TPE: 1-1.5 TPV; **IA:** 3 TPV   **Frequency—TPE:** daily; **IA:** daily

Replacement fluid—TPE: plasma; **IA:** NA

To remove inhibitors, plasma flow rates are 35 to 40 mL/minute in Immunosorba; a three-plasma-volume treatment (10 L) requires 20 to 30 adsorption cycles. Anticoagulant should be used at the lowest amount possible. These columns are not available in the United States. For inhibitors, procedures are performed daily until bleeding can be controlled with other therapeutic modalities.

(cont'd)

Table 1-6. Descriptions of Diseases for Which Therapeutic Apheresis Is Recommended* (Continued)

CRYOGLOBULINEMIA

Condition	Procedure	Recommendation	Category
Severe/symptomatic	TPE	Grade 2A	I
Severe/symptomatic	IA	Grade 2B	II

Volume treated: 1-1.5 TPV **Frequency:** every 1-3 days

Replacement fluid: albumin, plasma

It is prudent to warm the room, draw/return lines, and/or replacement fluid. There is a single case report of a patient receiving plasma exchange who developed acute oliguric renal failure due to infusion of cold plasma and precipitation of cryoglobulin within glomerular capillary loops. Other cases have reported cryoglobulin precipitation in the extracorporeal circuit.

The reports use a variety of treatments and frequencies. For acute symptoms, performance of three to eight procedures with reevaluation for clinical benefit should be considered. TPE may rapidly improve acute symptoms and serve as a bridging therapy before treating the underlying disease and reducing immunoglobulin production with immunosuppressive drugs. Weekly to monthly maintenance treatments may be indicated in patients who initially responded to TPE, in order to prevent recurrent symptoms. Because the cryocrit is not a marker of disease activity, it should not be used as a criterion for initiating or discontinuing TPE.

CUTANEOUS T-CELL LYMPHOMA (CTCL); MYCOSIS FUNGOIDES (MF); SEZARY SYNDROME (SS)

Condition	Procedure	Recommendation	Category
Erythrodermic	ECP	Grade 1B	I
Nonerythrodermic	ECP	Grade 2C	III

Volume treated: MNC product of 200-270 mL; the two-process method collects and treats MNCs obtained from two-TBV processing **Frequency:** 2 consecutive days (one cycle) every 2-4 weeks

Replacement fluid: NA

One cycle (two daily ECP procedures) once or twice per month yields comparable results to more frequent or intensive photopheresis regimens. For patients with SS, two monthly cycles have been recommended.

The median time for a maximal response to ECP is 5 to 6 months, although combination regimens may induce earlier remissions. Some patients may take as long as 10 months to respond. More rapid responses to ECP correlate with durability. Patients should be monitored and responses documented as per published guidelines. When maximal response is achieved with ECP, it can be reduced to one cycle every 6 to 12 weeks, with subsequent discontinuation if no relapses occur. If MF/SS recurs, ECP can be reinstituted at once or twice monthly. If there is no response or there is disease progression after 3 months of ECP alone, combination therapy or alternate agents should be considered.

(cont'd)

43

Table 1-6. Descriptions of Diseases for Which Therapeutic Apheresis Is Recommended* (Continued)

DILATED CARDIOMYOPATHY, IDIOPATHIC (IDCM)

Condition	Procedure	Recommendation	Category
NYHA II-IV	TPE	Grade 2C	III
NYHA II-IV	IA	Grade 1B	II

Volume treated—TPE: 1-1.5 TPV; **IA:** 2.5-5 L depending on the saturation and regeneration characteristics of the column

Replacement fluid—TPE: albumin; **IA:** NA

Frequency—TPE: five treatments daily or every other day; **IA:** various schedules, most commonly five treatments daily or every other day

Studies have examined only patients with symptoms for ≥6 months optimally medically managed. Patients with IDCM caused by inherited cytoskeletal abnormalities have not been treated and would not be expected to respond. Trials have used sheep antihuman immunoglobulin, staphylococcal protein A agarose (SPAA), and β1-adrenergic receptor extracellular domain columns. Comparison of these found SPAA less effective because of a lower affinity for pathogenic IgG3 antibodies. Modified SPAA protocols with enhanced IgG3 removal were effective. Retrospective comparison of the modified SPAA protocol and protocols using the recombinant β1-adrenergic receptor extracellular domain columns found equivalent response to therapy. An analysis comparing outcomes in patients with β1-adrenergic receptor antibody using specific IA vs nonspecific antibody removal found no difference in response or outcomes among the three IA columns examined (SPAA, recombinant β1-adrenergic receptor extracellular domain column, and immunoglobulin-binding peptide column). IVIG (0.5 g/kg) was given after the last apheresis treatment in the majority of IA studies and the TPE case series.

An IA trial comparing treatment consisting of a single course of 5 consecutive days to 4 courses of 5 consecutive days repeated every 4 weeks failed to demonstrate differences in left ventricular ejection fraction (LVEF) at 3 and 6 months between the two treatment schema. Repeat IA and TPE have been reported to be effective in patients experiencing increasing β1-adrenergic receptor antibody titers and/or worsening left ventricular ejection fraction.

45

(cont'd)

Table 1-6. Descriptions of Diseases for Which Therapeutic Apheresis Is Recommended* (Continued)

FAMILIAL HYPERCHOLESTEROLEMIA (FH)

Condition	Procedure	Recommendation	Category
Homozygotes (HM)*	LDL apheresis	Grade 1A	I
Heterozygotes (HT)	LDL apheresis	Grade 1A	II
Homozygotes with small blood volume†	TPE	Grade 1C	II

Volume treated—LDL apheresis: varies according to device; **Frequency:** adjusted to reduce the time-averaged LDL cholesterol **TPE:** 1-1.5 TPV by ≥60%, usually once every 1 to 2 weeks

Replacement fluid—LDL apheresis: NA; **TPE:** albumin

* Approved indications vary among countries; see below.
† Relative to manufacturer's recommendation for available selective removal devices.

Six selective removal systems are available: 1) immunoadsorption—columns containing matrix-bound sheep apoB antibodies; 2) dextran sulfate columns, which remove apoB lipoproteins from plasma by electrostatic interaction; 3) HELP, which precipitates apoB in the presence of heparin and low pH; 4) direct adsorption of lipoprotein using hemoperfusion, which removes apoB lipoproteins from whole blood through electrostatic interactions with polyacrylate-coated polyacrlyamide beads; 5) dextran sulfate cellulose columns—same mechanism as column in item 2 above, but treats whole blood; and 6) membrane differential filtration, which filters LDL from plasma. All have equivalent cholesterol reduction and side effects. Currently, the dextran sulfate plasma adsorption and HELP systems are cleared by the FDA.

ACE inhibitors are contraindicated in patients undergoing adsorption-based LDL apheresis. The columns function as a surface for plasma kallikrein generation, which converts bradykininogen to bradykinin. Kininase II inactivation of bradykinin is prevented by ACE inhibition, resulting in unopposed bradykinin effect, hypotension, and flushing. This is not seen with the HELP system.

Some LDL apheresis systems have been found to result in significant removal of vitamin B12, transferrin, and ferritin, which may cause anemia. Supplementation of vitamin B12 and iron may be necessary.

The goal is to reduce time-averaged total cholesterol >50% and LDL >60% from baseline. The time-averaged cholesterol can be calculated as follows: $C_{mean} = C_{min} + K(C_{max} - C_{min})$ where C_{mean} = the time-averaged cholesterol, C_{min} = the cholesterol level immediately after apheresis, K = the rebound coefficient, and C_{max} = the cholesterol level immediately before treatment. Values for K for FH HM and HT have been determined to be 0.65 and 0.71, respectively. To achieve these, reductions of total cholesterol of ≥65%, or LDL of ≥70%, must be achieved with each procedure. Numerous patient treatment criteria have been published. FDA criteria are 1) functional HM with LDL >500 mg/dL (>13 mmol/L); 2) functional HT with no known cardiovascular disease, but LDL ≥300 mg/dL (>7.8 mmol/L); and 3) functional HT with known cardiovascular disease and LDL ≥200 mg/dL (>5.2 mmol/L). The International Panel on Management of FH (Spain) indications are 1) FH HM and 2) HT patients with symptomatic coronary artery disease in whom LDL is >4.2 mmol/L (162 mg/dL) or decreases by <40% despite maximal medical management. The German Federal Committee of Physicians and Health Insurance Funds criteria are 1) FH HM and 2) patients with severe hypercholesterolemia in whom maximal dietary and drug therapy for >1 year has failed to lower cholesterol sufficiently. The HEART-UK criteria are 1) FH HM patients in whom LDL is reduced by <50% and/or >9 mmol/L (348 mg/dL) with drug therapy; 2) FH HT or a "bad family history" patients in whom LDL is reduced by <50% and/or >9 mmol/L (348 mg/dL) with drug therapy; or decreased by <40% despite drug therapy and drug therapy in whom LDL >5.0 mmol/L (193 mg/dL) or decreased by <40% despite drug with objective evidence of coronary disease progression and LDL >5.0 mmol/L

(cont'd)

Table 1-6. Descriptions of Diseases for Which Therapeutic Apheresis Is Recommended* (Continued)

therapy; and 3) progressive coronary artery disease, severe hypercholesterolemia, and Lp(a) >60 mg/dL (>3.3 mmol/L) in patients for whom LDL remains elevated despite drug therapy [see fact sheet on lipoprotein (a) hyperlipoproteinemia]. During pregnancy, LDL levels in individuals affected by FH can rise to extreme levels (1000 mg/dL (55 mmol/L)) that can compromise uteroplacental perfusion. There have been case reports of the use of LDL apheresis to allow for the successful completion of pregnancy.

TPE is effective, but the availability of the selective removal systems and their superior efficacy in cholesterol removal makes TPE use uncommon. TPE may be the only option in small children where the extracorporeal volume of selective removal systems is too large. It has been recommended that apheresis begin by age 6 or 7 to prevent aortic stenosis that can occur in homozygous FH. Treatment is continued indefinitely, adjusted to maintain the time-averaged cholesterol as described.

FOCAL SEGMENTAL GLOMERULOSCLEROSIS (FSGS)

Condition	Procedure	Recommendation	Category
Recurrent in transplanted kidney	TPE	Grade 1B	I

Volume treated: 1-1.5 TPV

Replacement fluid: albumin, plasma

Frequency: daily or every other day

Vascular access may be obtained through arteriovenous fistulas or grafts used for dialysis.

One approach is to begin with three daily TPEs, followed by at least six more TPEs in the subsequent 2 weeks, for a minimum of nine procedures. Another reported approach of intense/maintenance TPE treatment includes the following schedule: three per week for the first 3 weeks, followed by two TPEs per week for 3 weeks, one TPE per week until month 3, two TPEs per month until month 5, and once per month until month 9, but with concomitant immunosuppression treatment. Usually proteinuria decreases gradually while the patient is being treated with TPE as well as the creatinine, as reported in those patients who showed decreased renal clearance at diagnosis of FSGS recurrence. Tapering should be decided on a case-by-case basis and is guided by the degree of proteinuria. Timing of clinical response is quite variable, and complete abolishment of proteinuria may take several weeks to months. Some patients require long-term regimens of weekly to monthly TPEs to prevent reappearance of the proteinuria. There are no clinical or laboratory characteristics that predict the likelihood of success with TPE. Although the optimum timing of initiating TPE has not been studied, it is recommended that TPE be instituted as soon as recurrent FSGS is diagnosed, in order to halt the process and maintain kidney function.

(cont'd)

Table 1-6. Descriptions of Diseases for Which Therapeutic Apheresis Is Recommended* (Continued)

GRAFT-VS-HOST DISEASE (GVHD)

Condition	Procedure	Recommendation	Category
Skin (chronic)	ECP	Grade 1B	II
Skin (acute)	ECP	Grade 1C	II
Non-skin	ECP	Grade 2B	III

Volume treated: MNC product of 200-270 mL; the two-process method collects and treats MNCs obtained from two-TBV processing

Frequency: 2 consecutive days (one cycle) every 1-2 weeks

Replacement fluid: NA

ECP in individuals ≥40 kg can be performed using an intermittent-flow system (UVAR XTS photopheresis system). The CELLEX instrument (Therakos, Raritan, NJ) uses a continuous-flow system allowing treatment of patients ≥22 kg or smaller, by incorporating a blood prime. Heparin is the conventional anticoagulant for Therakos instruments, but ACD-A can be substituted if necessary. An alternative two-process method is commonly used in Europe and for smaller-body-weight patients (ie, <40 kg or when the extracorporeal volume exceeds 15% at any time during the collection or processing of the blood). This involves collecting MNCs by standard continuous-flow apheresis, photoactivating the MNCs by using a UVA light box (not approved in the United States), and reinfusing the treated cells.

For acute GVHD, one cycle is performed weekly until disease response and then tapered to every other week before discontinuation. For chronic GVHD, one cycle should be performed weekly (or consider biweekly if treating only mucocutaneous chronic GVHD) either until a response or for 8 to 12 weeks, followed by a taper to every 2 to 4 weeks until maximal response.

50

HEMATOPOIETIC STEM CELL TRANSPLANTATION, ABO INCOMPATIBLE

Condition	Procedure	Recommendation	Category
Major HPC(M)	TPE	Grade 1B	II
Major HPC(A)	TPE	Grade 2B	II
Minor HPC(A)	RBC exchange	Grade 2C	III

Volume treated—TPE: 1-2 TPV; **RBC exchange:** **Frequency:** daily
1-1.5 RBC volumes

Replacement fluid—TPE: albumin, or albumin and donor-and-recipient-ABO-compatible plasma; **RBC exchange:** group O RBCs

HPC(A) = HPC, apheresis; HPC(M) = HPC, marrow; major = major ABO incompatibility; minor = minor ABO incompatibility.

TPE should be performed before infusion of major ABO-incompatible HPC product, using albumin or a combination of albumin and plasma compatible with both donor and recipient as replacement fluid. Automated red cell exchange has involved exchanging 1 to 1.5 times the patient's red cell volume with group O RBCs.

For major incompatibility, the goal is to reduce the IgM or IgG antibody titers to ≤16 immediately before HPC transplantation. If there is a delayed red cell recovery or pure red cell aplasia (PRCA), TPE may be performed (see fact sheet on PRCA). For high-risk patients undergoing minor-incompatible transplantation, RBC exchange to 35% residual host erythrocytes is recommended.

(cont'd)

51

Table 1-6. Descriptions of Diseases for Which Therapeutic Apheresis Is Recommended* (Continued)

HEMOLYTIC UREMIC SYNDROME, ATYPICAL (AHUS)

Condition	Procedure	Recommendation	Category
Complement factor gene mutations	TPE	Grade 2C	II
Factor H autoantibodies	TPE	Grade 2C	I
Membrane cofactor protein mutations	TPE	Grade 1C	IV

Volume treated: 1-1.5 TPV   **Frequency:** daily

Replacement fluid: plasma; albumin (T-activation-associated HUS)

Because the majority of affected patients with aHUS are children, establishment of vascular access, RBC prime, and calcium supplementation are of special concern.

Because there is no standardized approach, the duration and schedule of TPE for treatment of TTP have been empirically adopted to treat aHUS. European Group recommends that TPE be performed daily for 5 days after urgent initiation of TPE, five times per week for 2 weeks, then three times per week for 2 weeks, with outcome evaluated at day 33. These guidelines address neither continued treatment after initial therapy failure nor ongoing prophylactic treatment for patients with remission. As shown in a recent case series of three patients with *CFH* mutation, acute and prophylactic TPE in the pre- and post-renal-transplant periods were effective in maintaining long-term native and allograft kidney function. Decisions regarding duration or discontinuation should be made based on patient response and condition.

HEMOLYTIC UREMIC SYNDROME (HUS), INFECTION ASSOCIATED

Condition	Procedure	Recommendation	Category
STEC-HUS	TPE	Grade 1C	IV
pHUS	TPE	Grade 2C	III

Volume treated: 1-1.5 TPV **Frequency:** daily

Replacement fluid—STEC-HUS: plasma; **pHUS:** albumin

pHUS = HUS associated with *Streptococcus pneumonia*; STEC-HUS = HUS associated with Shiga-toxin-producing *Escherichia coli*.

When TPE is performed in children with pHUS, avoidance of plasma-containing blood components is recommended to prevent the passive transfer of anti-T in normal plasma and possible polyagglutination caused by T activation. One longitudinal study of over 110 HUS/TTP patients has indicated that increased daily volumes of plasma may be associated with improved outcomes.

Because there is no standardized approach, the duration and schedule of TPE for treatment of TTP have been empirically adopted to treat HUS. Decisions regarding duration or discontinuation should be made based on patient response and condition.

(cont'd)

Table 1-6. Descriptions of Diseases for Which Therapeutic Apheresis Is Recommended* (Continued)

HENOCH-SCHÖNLEIN PURPURA (HSP)

Condition	Procedure	Recommendation	Category
Crescentic	TPE	Grade 2C	III
Severe extrarenal manifestations	TPE	Grade 2C	III

Volume treated: 1-1.5 TPV **Frequency:** 4-11 over 21 days
Replacement fluid: albumin

Replacement fluid has varied depending on the clinical situation, with the final portion consisting of plasma in the presence of intracranial hemorrhage in cerebritis or GI bleeding. Double-filtration plasmapheresis has also been used in a single patient with RPGN in HSP, with resolution of renal disease.

In cerebritis and severe GI manifestations, the course of therapy has ranged from one to six TPEs daily, with discontinuation of TPE upon resolution of symptoms. In RPGN, longer courses of therapy have occurred, and therapy was discontinued with improvement in renal function as determined by creatinine measurement.

HEPARIN-INDUCED THROMBOCYTOPENIA (HIT)

Condition	Procedure	Recommendation	Category
Pre-CPB	TPE	Grade 2C	III
Thrombosis	TPE	Grade 2C	III

Volume treated: 1-1.5 TPV   **Frequency:** daily or every other day

Replacement fluid: albumin, plasma

CPB = cardiopulmonary bypass.

Because a high percentage of cardiac surgery patients have heparin-PF4-directed antibodies as detected by ELISA (a highly sensitive but relatively nonspecific assay), the diagnosis of HIT must be based on high clinical suspicion as determined by one of two scoring systems [4T score or the HIT expert probability (HEP) score]. A confirmatory functional platelet activation assay, the serotonin release assay (SRA), may be helpful in the complex patient. In the absence of access to the SRA assay, the potential risks and benefits of performing TPE followed by intraoperative heparin use in place of unfractionated heparin alone (without pre-CPB TPE) or alternative anticoagulation should involve a careful evaluation of the HIT score and results of HIT testing (eg, ELISA/HIPA). If TPE is used, the laboratory must be able to reliably quantitate the HIT antibody titer as a guide to TPE efficacy (as outlined below).

In the setting of CPB, TPE has typically been used preoperatively until HIT antibody titers become negative by the testing method used. In the setting of thrombosis, the number of procedures performed in clinical reports has been guided by clinical response (eg, resolution of thrombosis-related tissue ischemia) and reduction in HIT-antibody levels with TPE (conversion of positive to negative result in the HIT assay).

(cont'd)

Table 1-6. Descriptions of Diseases for Which Therapeutic Apheresis Is Recommended* (Continued)

HEREDITARY HEMOCHROMATOSIS

Procedure	Recommendation	Category
Erythrocytapheresis	Grade 1B	I
Volume treated: erythrocytapheresis of up to 800 mL of RBCs		**Frequency:** every 2-3 weeks, keeping the preprocedure Hct ≥34% and postprocedure Hct ≥30%
Replacement fluid: replace at least one-third to one-half of removed RBC volume with saline		

Although reported methods vary, the Dutch trial employed a schedule of erythrocytapheresis of 350 to 800 mL of erythrocytes every 2 weeks. The preprocedure hemoglobin should be ≥12 mg/dL or Hct ≥34%. An interval of 3 weeks may be required, especially for women, to avoid a postprocedure Hct <30%. The actual volume of erythrocytes to be removed (VR) with each procedure can be calculated as follows:

$$VR = [(\text{starting Hct} - \text{target Hct}) \div 79] \times [\text{blood volume (mL/kg)} \times \text{body weight (kg)}]$$

Erythrocytapheresis should be performed every 2 to 3 weeks, or as tolerated, until serum ferritin <50 ng/mL. Maintenance treatment can follow with infrequent therapeutic phlebotomy or erythrocytapheresis.

56

HYPERLEUKOCYTOSIS

Condition	Procedure	Recommendation	Category
Leukostasis	Leukocytapheresis	Grade 1B	I
Prophylaxis	Leukocytapheresis	Grade 2C	III

Volume treated: 1.5-2 TBV

Replacement fluid: crystalloid; albumin, plasma

Frequency: daily; twice-daily for life-threatening cases

A single procedure can reduce the WBC count by 30% to 60%. Erythrocyte-sedimenting agents (eg, hydroxyethyl starch) are not required for acute myeloid leukemia (AML) or acute lymphoid leukemia (ALL). Red cell priming may be employed for selected adults with severe anemia; however, undiluted packed RBCs should be avoided in small children with hyperviscosity. Replacement fluid should be used to ensure at least a net even ending fluid balance of ± 15% of TBV. The collection rate at the start of and during the procedure should be carefully adjusted and monitored to optimize WBC removal and ensure safety.

Treatments should be discontinued: 1) for prophylaxis of asymptomatic AML patients, when the blast cell count is <100 × 10^9/L (closely monitor patients with M4 and M5 subtypes); 2) for AML patients with leukostasis complications, when the blast cell count is <50 to 100 × 10^9/L and clinical manifestations have resolved; 3) for prophylaxis of asymptomatic ALL patients, when the blast cell count is <400 × 10^9/L; and 4) for those with leukostasis complications, when the blast cell count is <400 × 10^9/L and clinical manifestations have resolved.

(cont'd)

57

Table 1-6. Descriptions of Diseases for Which Therapeutic Apheresis Is Recommended* (Continued)

HYPERTRIGLYCERIDEMIC (HTG) PANCREATITIS

Procedure	Recommendation	Category
TPE	Grade 2C	III
Volume treated: 1-1.5 TPV	**Frequency—therapeutic:** daily for 1-3 days depending on patient course and triglyceride (TG) level; **prophylactic:** every 2-4 weeks to maintain TG level below 150 mg/dL	
Replacement fluid: albumin, plasma		

Both centrifugal and double-membrane filtration TPE have been used to treat pancreatitis from HTG. A comparison of these two methods found greater removal with centrifugal methods, because of the tendency of the TG to clog the pores of the filters.

Reports have suggested that heparin should be used as the anticoagulant for these procedures because of its ability to release lipoprotein lipase (LPL), which should enhance TG reduction. Many reports have used ACD-A with similar TG reductions. Most reports have used albumin as the replacement fluid. Some have used plasma, as it contains LPL and could enhance TG removal. No direct comparisons of anticoagulants or replacement fluids have been reported. Treatment has usually been implemented early in the course of the pancreatitis secondary to HTG, although some authors have recommended its use only if there is no improvement with standard therapy.

For patients with acute pancreatitis, one TPE has been sufficient to improve the patient's clinical condition and lower the TG levels, with additional treatments if necessary. For patients treated prophylactically, chronic therapy for years has been reported.

HYPERVISCOSITY IN MONOCLONAL GAMMOPATHIES

Condition	Procedure	Recommendation	Category
Symptomatic	TPE	Grade 1B	I
Prophylaxis for rituximab	TPE	Grade 1C	I

Volume treated: 1-1.5 TPV **Frequency**: daily
Replacement fluid: albumin

There is no uniform consensus regarding the preferred exchange volume for treatment of hyperviscosity. It is understood that viscosity falls rapidly as M-protein is removed; thus, relatively small exchange volumes are effective. Conventional calculations of plasma volume based on weight and Hct are inaccurate in M-protein disorders because of plasma volume expansion. Therefore, an empirical exchange of 1 to 1.5 plasma volumes per procedure seems reasonable. A direct comparison trial demonstrated that centrifugation apheresis is more efficient than cascade filtration in removing M-protein. Cascade filtration and membrane filtration techniques have been described in case reports, but most American institutions employ continuous-centrifugation plasma exchange.

Patients can be treated daily until acute symptoms abate (generally one to three procedures). At that point, serum viscosity measurement can be repeated to determine the point at which the patient experiences symptomatic hyperviscosity relief. Retinal changes in otherwise asymptomatic patients with Waldenström macroglobulinemia respond dramatically to a single plasma exchange, with marked or complete reversal of the abnormal findings. An empirical maintenance schedule of 1 plasma volume exchange every 1 to 4 weeks based on clinical symptoms or retinal changes may be used to maintain clinical stability pending a salutary effect of medical therapy (eg, chemotherapy, targeted therapy, etc). Prophylactic TPE to lower IgM to <5000 mg/dL may be performed in preparation for a treatment regimen that includes rituximab.

(cont'd)

59

Table 1-6. Descriptions of Diseases for Which Therapeutic Apheresis Is Recommended* (Continued)

IMMUNE COMPLEX RAPIDLY PROGRESSIVE GLOMERULONEPHRITIS

Procedure	Recommendation	Category
TPE	Grade 2B	III
Volume treated: 1-1.5 TPV	**Frequency:** every other day	
Replacement fluid: albumin		

TPE may be beneficial in dialysis-dependent patients at presentation.

Treatment for 1 to 2 weeks should be followed by tapering to less frequent treatments. The duration of therapy is not well defined in the literature. Some trials have stopped TPE if there is no response after 4 weeks of therapy as outlined above.

IMMUNE THROMBOCYTOPENIA (ITP)

Condition	Procedure	Recommendation	Category
Refractory	TPE	Grade 2C	IV
Refractory	IA	Grade 2C	III

Volume treated—IA: 1000-2000 mL plasma online;
250-500 mL plasma off-line

Frequency—IA: once a week or every 2-3 days

Replacement fluid—IA: NA

Using staphylococcal protein A silica, the procedure can be performed either online after separation of plasma by continuous-flow cell separator or off-line using phlebotomized blood. Plasma is treated by perfusion through the column and then reinfused with a flow rate not exceeding 20 mL/minute. No significant difference between the two methods has been demonstrated in either safety or effectiveness. In children, extra care must be given to maintain isovolemia because of the large extracorporeal volume involved with the procedure.

There are no clear guidelines concerning treatment schedule and duration of treatment. The procedure is generally discontinued when the patient shows either improvement in platelet count ($>50 \times 10^9$/L) or no improvement after about six treatments.

(cont'd)

Table 1-6. Descriptions of Diseases for Which Therapeutic Apheresis Is Recommended* (Continued)

IMMUNOGLOBIN A NEPHROPATHY

Condition	Procedure	Recommendation	Category
Crescentic	TPE	Grade 2B	III
Chronic progressive	TPE	Grade 2C	III

Volume treated: 1-1.5 TPV
Replacement fluid: albumin

Frequency: six to nine treatments over 21 days followed by three to six over 6 weeks

The greatest benefit appears to occur in those patients with RPGN and in whom renal biopsy demonstrates cellular crescents. Response appears unlikely to occur in chronic disease, if biopsy demonstrates sclerotic glomeruli, or if there is delay in starting TPE following onset of acute kidney failure.

A fixed course of therapy has been used to treat patients presenting with RPGN. Creatinine is monitored to determine response. In chronic progressive disease, chronic therapy with weekly TPE for up to 4 months has been reported.

INFLAMMATORY BOWEL DISEASE

Condition	Procedure	Recommendation	Category
UC	Adsorptive cytapheresis	Grade 1B*/2B†	III*/II†
CD	Adsorptive cytapheresis	Grade 1B	II
CD	ECP	Grade 2C	III

Volume treated—Adacolumn: 1800 mL

Cellsorba: 3000 mL

Replacement fluid: NA

Frequency: once per week; more intensive therapy may include daily treatment twice per week

CD = Crohn disease; UC = ulcerative colitis.
*The standard of care in the United States includes immunosuppression with tumor necrosis factor (TNF)α blockade.
†Conventional therapy in Asia consists of steroids and aminosalicylates alone.
It is possible that the above accounts for positive outcomes for adsorptive cytotherapy found in Asian, but not North American, studies.

Two types of selective apheresis devices are the Cellsorba (Asahi Medical, Tokyo, Japan), which is a column containing cylindrical nonwoven polyester fibers, and the Adacolumn (JIMRO, Takasaki, Japan), which contains cellulose acetate beads. Both require anticoagulation (heparin/ACD-A and heparin alone, respectively) to remove granulocytes and monocytes from venous whole blood by filtration/adhesion. For Cellsorba, venous whole blood is processed at 50 mL/minute through the column for 60 minutes. Some platelets and lymphocytes are also removed by this column. For Adacolumn, venous whole blood is processed at 30 mL/minute for

(cont'd)

63

Table 1-6. Descriptions of Diseases for Which Therapeutic Apheresis Is Recommended* (Continued)

60 minutes. The Adacolumn is relatively selective for removing activated granulocytes and monocytes. Patients taking ACE inhibitors may experience low blood pressure if undergoing treatment with Adacolumn. Cellsorba and Adacolumn are currently available in Europe and Japan. The two columns have been compared in a prospective clinical trial that demonstrated equivalent response in patients with moderate-to-severe active UC.

The typical length of treatment is 5 to 10 weeks for Adacolumn, and 5 weeks for Cellsorba.

LAMBERT-EATON MYASTHENIC SYNDROME

Procedure	Recommendation	Category
TPE	Grade 2C	II
Volume treated: 1-1.5 TPV	**Frequency:** daily or every other day	
Replacement fluid: albumin		

The reported TPE regimens vary from 5 to 15 daily TPEs over 5 to 19 days, to 8 to 10 TPEs carried out at 5- to 7-day intervals. Most reports indicate an exchange volume of 1.25 plasma volumes. Of note, improvement may not be seen for the 2 weeks or more after initiation of TPE. This may result from the slower turnover of the presynaptic voltage-gated calcium channel compared to the post-synaptic acetylcholine receptor.

Treatment should continue until a clear clinical and electromyogram response is obtained, or at least until a 2- to 3-week course of TPE has been completed. Repeated courses may be applied in case of neurologic relapse, but the effect can be expected to last only 2 to 4 weeks in the absence of immunosuppressive drug therapy.

(cont'd)

Table 1-6. Descriptions of Diseases for Which Therapeutic Apheresis Is Recommended* (Continued)

LIPOPROTEIN (A) HYPERLIPOPROTEINEMIA

Procedure	Recommendation	Category
LDL apheresis	Grade 1B	II

Volume treated: varies according to device **Frequency:** once every 1-2 weeks
Replacement fluid: NA

The six available LDL apheresis devices (see *familial hypercholesterolemia*) are all capable of removing Lp(a) with similar degrees of reduction. There have been no reports of the use of TPE to treat elevations of Lp(a).

ACE inhibitors are contraindicated in patients undergoing adsorption-based LDL apheresis. The columns function as a surface for plasma kallikrein generation, which in turn converts bradykininogen to bradykinin. Kininase II inactivation of bradykinin is prevented by ACE inhibition, resulting in unopposed bradykinin effect, hypotension, and flushing. This is not seen with the HELP system.

Some LDL apheresis systems have also been found to result in significant removal of vitamin B12, transferrin, and ferritin. This may be the cause of the anemia seen in patients undergoing therapy, and supplementation may be necessary.

The European Atherosclerosis Society Consensus Panel recommends the reduction of Lp(a) to less than the 80th percentile of normal, <50 mg/dL (2.77 mmol/L). The HEART-UK criteria for the use of LDL apheresis includes patients with progressive coronary artery disease, hypercholesterolemia, and Lp(a) >60 mg/dL (>3.3 mmol/L), in whom LDL cholesterol remains elevated despite drug therapy. Other LDL apheresis treatment criteria, such as those published by the FDA, International Panel on Management of Familial Hypercholesterolemia, and the German Federal Committee of Physicians and Health Insurance Funds, do not include Lp(a) in their criteria for LDL apheresis. However, in Germany, LDL apheresis is used in Lp(a) hyperlipoproteinemia in the presence of progressive coronary artery disease and failure of drug therapy.

Treatment is continued indefinitely, adjusted to maintain the Lp(a) below 50 mg/dL (2.77 mmol/L).

(cont'd)

Table 1-6. Descriptions of Diseases for Which Therapeutic Apheresis Is Recommended* (Continued)

LIVER TRANSPLANTATION, ABO INCOMPATIBLE (ABOi)

Condition	Procedure	Recommendation	Category
Desensitization (LDLT)	TPE	Grade 1C	I
Desensitization (DDLT)	TPE	Grade 2C	III
Humoral rejection	TPE	Grade 2C	III

Volume treated: 1-1.5 TPV **Frequency:** daily or every other day

Replacement fluid: albumin, plasma

LDLT = live-donor liver transplant; DDLT = deceased-donor liver transplant.

The replacement fluid for TPE is plasma, or albumin and plasma (plasma should be compatible with both the recipient and donor). Plasma use may need to be more aggressive in the setting of ABOi liver transplantation because of coagulopathy secondary to liver failure in the recipient.

The goal should be to reduce the antibody titer to less than a critical threshold before taking the patient to transplantation. It is important to note that this critical titer will need to be determined by each program embarking on this type of transplant, given that titer results can vary widely depending on titration method and technique. The number of TPE procedures required depends on the patient's baseline ABO titer and on the rate of antibody production/rebound. Unlike in ABOi renal transplantation, the predictive value of posttransplant titers is less-well established. Patients should be monitored closely for graft function before discontinuation of TPE.

LUNG ALLOGRAFT REJECTION

Condition	Procedure	Recommendation	Category
Bronchiolitis obliterans syndrome	ECP	Grade 1C	II
	TPE	Grade 2C	III
Antibody-mediated rejection			

Volume treated—ECP: MNC product of 200-270 mL; the two-process method collects and treats MNCs obtained from two-TBV processing; **TPE:** 1-1.5 PV

Replacement fluid—ECP: NA; **TPE:** albumin, plasma

Frequency—ECP: see above; **TPE:** daily or every other day

In the largest case series of ECP in bronchiolitis obliterans syndrome, 24 ECP treatments were administered during a 6-month period, delivered as two treatments on successive days. Ten treatments were performed over the first month, followed biweekly for the next 2 months (eight treatments), and then monthly for the remaining 3 months (six treatments).

The optimal duration of treatment is not well established. If clinical stabilization occurs with ECP, long-term continuation may be warranted to maintain the clinical response. In a recent 10-year single-center experience, 24 treatments were the initial "dose," and long-term continuation (two treatments per month) was recommended for responders. For pulmonary antibody-mediated rejection, TPE treatment may be discontinued, with reversal of rejection as evidenced by an improvement in allograft function or reduction in donor-specific antibody levels.

(cont'd)

Table 1-6. Descriptions of Diseases for Which Therapeutic Apheresis Is Recommended* (Continued)

MALARIA

Condition	Procedure	Recommendation	Category
Severe	RBC exchange	Grade 2B	II

Volume treated: 1-2 total RBC volumes **Frequency:** usually one to two treatments

Replacement fluid: RBCs (consider leukocyte-reduced), plasma

Automated apheresis instruments calculate the amount of RBCs required to achieve the desired postprocedure Hct, fraction of red cells remaining, and, by inference, the estimated final parasite load. A single two-volume RBC exchange can reduce the fraction of remaining patient red cells to roughly 10% to 15% of the original. The risks include circulatory overload, transfusion reactions, blood-borne infection (especially in developing countries), hypocalcemia, red cell allosensitization, and possible need for central venous access.

  Treatment is discontinued after achieving significant clinical improvement and/or <1% residual parasitemia.

MULTIPLE SCLEROSIS (MS)

Condition	Procedure	Recommendation	Category
Acute CNS inflammatory demyelinating	TPE	Grade 1B	II
Disease unresponsive to steroids	IA	Grade 2C	III
Chronic progressive	TPE	Grade 2B	III

Volume treated: 1-1.5 TPV

Replacement fluid: albumin

Frequency—acute: five to seven over 14 days; **chronic progressive:** weekly

In acute MS relapse unresponsive to steroids, five to seven TPE procedures have a response rate of approximately 50%. Studies have found that early initiation of therapy, within 14 to 20 days of onset of symptoms, is a predictor of response. However, response still occurred in patients treated 60 days after the onset of symptoms. In chronic progressive MS, TPE could be a long-term therapy, if shown to be of benefit, with tapering as tolerated.

(cont'd)

Table 1-6. Descriptions of Diseases for Which Therapeutic Apheresis Is Recommended* (Continued)

MYASTHENIA GRAVIS

Condition	Procedure	Recommendation	Category
Moderate to severe	TPE	Grade 1B	I
Prethymectomy	TPE	Grade 1C	I

Volume treated: 1-1.5 TPV
Replacement fluid: albumin
Frequency: daily or every other day

A typical induction regimen consists of processing 225 mL/kg of plasma over a period of up to 2 weeks, but smaller-volume processing can be beneficial. The number and frequency of procedures depends on the clinical scenario. Some patients may require long-term maintenance TPE.

MYELOMA CAST NEPHROPATHY

Procedure	Recommendation	Category
TPE	Grade 2B	II

Volume treated: 1-1.5 TPV **Frequency:** daily or every other day
Replacement fluid: albumin

Initial management, especially in the case of nonoliguric patients, should focus on fluid resuscitation (2.5-4 liters/day), alkaliniza-tion of the urine, and chemotherapy. If serum creatinine remains elevated after several days, addition of plasma exchange should be considered. For oliguric patients who excrete ≥10 grams of light chains every 24 hours, or whose serum creatinine is ≥6 mg/dL, plasma exchange may be included in initial management, especially in the case of light-chain myeloma. All of the published studies combine TPE with chemotherapy and other forms of supportive care described above. Published studies vary with respect to treat-ment schedules and replacement fluids employed for TPE. If TPE and hemodialysis are to be performed on the same day, they can be performed in tandem (simultaneously) without compromising the efficiency of the hemodialysis procedure.

Controlled trials have used TPE as a short-term adjunct to chemotherapy and fluid resuscitation over a period of 2 to 4 weeks. In some studies and reports, a course of plasma exchange (10-12 procedures over 2-3 weeks) may be repeated depending on the patient's clinical course.

(cont'd)

73

Table 1-6. Descriptions of Diseases for Which Therapeutic Apheresis Is Recommended* (Continued)

NEPHROGENIC SYSTEMIC FIBROSIS

Procedure	Recommendation	Category
ECP	Grade 2C	III
TPE	Grade 2C	III

Volume treated—ECP: MNC product typically obtained after processing 1.5 L of blood (CELLEX/UVAR XTS); The two-step method collects and treats MNCs obtained from two-TBV processing; **TPE:** 1-1.5 TPV

Replacement fluid—ECP: NA; **TPE:** albumin

Frequency—ECP: various schedules ranging from two procedures in consecutive days every 2-4 weeks, up to five every other day (cycle), with an increasing number of weeks between cycles (1-4), and 4 cycles composing a round; **TPE:** various schedules ranging from daily for five treatments to twice per week for 10 to 14 treatments

The relationship between time of initiation of therapy and reversal of changes is unclear. Whether the changes become irreversible and whether earlier treatment is more effective than later treatment have not been determined.

The time to response has not been reported for most patients treated with TPE. Improvement of early symptoms in one patient was reported to have occurred within 3 days of initiation of treatment. The time to response with ECP ranged from 4 to 16 months. Reports have treated patients for a fixed number of procedures.

NEUROMYELITIS OPTICA (NMO)

Condition	Procedure	Recommendation	Category
Acute	TPE	Grade 1B	II
Maintenance	TPE	Grade 2C	III

Volume treated: 1-1.5 TPV
Replacement fluid: albumin

Frequency—acute: daily or every other day; **maintenance:** variable

Double-filtration plasmapheresis has also been reported as successful for controlling NMO exacerbation.

The majority of studies performed five procedures on average for acute NMO exacerbation, but ranged from two to 20 procedures.

In one case series, five out of seven patients who were on maintenance TPE therapy (three per week for 2 weeks, two per week for 2 weeks, then weekly for 3-5 weeks) showed varying degrees of improvement and reduction in the number of NMO exacerbations.

(cont'd)

Table 1-6. Descriptions of Diseases for Which Therapeutic Apheresis Is Recommended* (Continued)

OVERDOSE, ENVENOMATION, AND POISONING

Condition	Procedure	Recommendation	Category
Mushroom poisoning	TPE	Grade 2C	II
Envenomation	TPE	Grade 2C	III
Natalizumab/PML	TPE	Grade 2C	III
Tacrolimus	RBC exchange	Grade 2C	III

Volume treated: 1 to 2 TPV **Frequency:** daily

Replacement fluid: albumin, plasma

PML = progressive multifocal leukoencephalopathy.

The replacement fluid chosen should be one that contains enough protein to draw toxin into the blood compartment for elimination; albumin is such an agent and generally acts as an effective replacement fluid. However, some toxic substances may bind to other plasma constituents preferentially over albumin. For example, dipyridamole, quinidine, imipramine, propranolol, and chlorpromazine are known to have strong affinity for alpha-1-acid glycoprotein; for overdoses of these agents, plasma may be a more appropriate choice. Some venoms also cause coagulopathy and possibly microangiopathy with low levels of ADAMTS13, in which case the use of plasma should be strongly considered.

TPEs are usually performed and continued on a daily basis until the clinical symptoms have abated, and delayed release of toxin from tissues is no longer problematic.

PARANEOPLASTIC NEUROLOGIC SYNDROMES

Procedure	Recommendation	Category
TPE	Grade 2C	III
IA	Grade 2C	III

Volume treated—TPE: 1-1.5 TPV; **IA:** 500-1000 mL of plasma   **Frequency—TPE:** daily or every other day;
Replacement fluid—TPE: albumin; **IA:** NA   **IA:** twice weekly

TPE cannot be considered standard therapy for autoimmune paraneoplastic neurologic syndromes. Protein A immunoadsorption, either "online" or "off-line," may be employed, particularly for paraneoplastic opsoclonus/myoclonus, although there is very little published experience.

Duration of procedures is usually five to six procedures over up to 2 weeks for TPE, and twice weekly for 3 weeks for protein A immunoadsorption.

(cont'd)

Table 1-6. Descriptions of Diseases for Which Therapeutic Apheresis Is Recommended* (Continued)

PARAPROTEINEMIC DEMYELINATING NEUROPATHIES

Condition	Procedure	Recommendation	Category
IgG/IgA	TPE	Grade 1B	I
IgM	TPE	Grade 1C	I
Multiple myeloma	TPE	Grade 2C	III
IgG/IgA/IgM	IA	Grade 2C	III

Volume treated: 1-1.5 TPV   **Frequency:** every other day
Replacement fluid: albumin, plasma

Patients with demyelinating paraproteinemia may be treated at any time in their course (including patients referred up to 4 years after onset of symptoms).

The typical course is five to six treatments over the course of 10 to 14 days. Long-term TPE or slow tapering off of TPE can be considered. The patient may continue to improve over the weeks following cessation of plasma exchange. If the level of paraprotein is correlative to the polyneuropathy, it can be monitored to evaluate the frequency of treatment. However, the titer of the paraprotein may not correlate with the clinical disease state.

PEDIATRIC AUTOIMMUNE NEUROPSYCHIATRIC DISORDERS ASSOCIATED WITH STREPTOCOCCAL INFECTIONS (PANDAS); SYDENHAM CHOREA (SC)

Condition	Procedure	Recommendation	Category
PANDAS, exacerbation	TPE	Grade 1B	I
SC	TPE	Grade 1B	I

Volume treated: 1-1.5 TPV   **Frequency**: daily or every other day
Replacement fluid: albumin

Five or six procedures over 7 to 14 days were used in the RCT. There are no data on any benefit of repeated treatment.

(cont'd)

Table 1-6. Descriptions of Diseases for Which Therapeutic Apheresis Is Recommended* (Continued)

PEMPHIGUS VULGARIS

Condition	Procedure	Recommendation	Category
Severe	TPE	Grade 2B	III
Severe	ECP	Grade 2C	III
Severe	IA	Grade 2C	III

Volume treated—TPE: 1-1.5 TPV; **ECP:** MNC product of 200-270 mL; the two-process method collects and treats MNCs obtained from two-TBV processing.

IA: per manufacturers' recommendations

Frequency—TPE: daily or every other day; **ECP:** 2 consecutive days (one series) every 2 or 4 weeks; **IA:** daily up to 4 days and followed up by various frequency protocols

Replacement fluid—TPE: albumin, plasma; **ECP:** NA; **IA:** NA

The TPE protocols used in pemphigus vulgaris vary widely and usually have been based on the observed clinical response after each treatment. The reported volumes processed have been as low as 400 mL and as high as 4000 mL, and the reported frequency of treatments has varied widely as well. However, more recent reports noted that one-plasma-volume exchanges are preferable in patients who are resistant to conventional therapy. The levels of autoantibody have been noted to rebound in the reported patients within 1 to 2 weeks after discontinuation of treatment, which necessitates continuation of immunosuppression. The clinical response in patients who underwent ECP was observed after two to seven cycles (two daily procedures per cycle). The total number of cycles received varied from 2 to 48. In one report, 100% clinical response with decreased autoantibody titer was reported.

The follow-up ranged between 4 and 48 months. The disease was controlled in most patients, but only two patients were able to discontinue all oral systemic agents.

For TPE and IA, as noted above, the treatment protocols are highly variable. The rational approach should include monitoring of autoantibody titers and clinical symptoms. The lack of clinical response after a trial period with concomitant adequate immunosuppression should be sufficient to discontinue treatment.

For ECP, the treatments were continued until clinical response was noted. The rational discontinuation criteria should be similar to those for TPE.

(cont'd)

81

Table 1-6. Descriptions of Diseases for Which Therapeutic Apheresis Is Recommended* (Continued)

PERIPHERAL VASCULAR DISEASES

Procedure	Recommendation	Category
LDL apheresis	Grade 2C	III

Volume treated: 3000-5000 mL of plasma volume

Replacement fluid: NA

Frequency: once or twice per week

Six selective removal systems are available: 1) immunoadsorption—columns containing matrix-bound sheep apoB antibodies; 2) dextran sulfate columns, which remove apoB-containing lipoproteins from plasma by electrostatic interaction; 3) HELP, which precipitates apoB molecules in the presence of heparin and low pH; 4) direct adsorption of lipoprotein using hemoperfusion, which removes apoB lipoproteins from whole blood through electrostatic interactions with polyacrylate-coated polyacrlyamide beads; 5) dextran sulfate cellulose columns, which remove apoB-containing lipoproteins from whole blood through electrostatic interactions; and 6) membrane differential filtration, which filters LDL from plasma. All have equivalent cholesterol reduction and side effects. Currently, the dextran sulfate plasma adsorption and HELP systems are approved by the FDA.

ACE inhibitors are contraindicated in patients undergoing adsorption-based LDL apheresis. The columns function as a surface for plasma kallikrein generation, which converts bradykininogen to bradykinin. Kininase II inactivation of bradykinin is prevented by ACE inhibition, resulting in unopposed bradykinin effect, hypotension, and flushing. This is not seen with the HELP system.

Ten treatments in less than an 8-week period have been used.

PHYTANIC ACID (PA) STORAGE DISEASE (REFSUM DISEASE)

Procedure	Recommendation	Category
TPE	Grade 2C	II
LDL apheresis	Grade 2C	II

Volume treated—TPE: 1-1.5 TPV; **LDL apheresis:** 3 L
Replacement fluid—TPE: albumin; **LDL apheresis:** NA

Frequency: daily for acute exacerbation; variable for chronic therapy

Although approaches to therapeutic apheresis for Refsum disease vary, a typical course consists of one to two TPEs per week for several weeks to a month. In some cases, maintenance plasma exchanges continue with decreasing frequency over subsequent weeks to months. When LDL apheresis has been used for chronic therapy, treatments have been given weekly to every other week.

Therapeutic strategy is ultimately determined by monitoring the patient's PA level and clinical signs and symptoms, and the need to control or prevent exacerbations of the disease. If chronic therapy is initiated, procedures should be performed lifelong.

(cont'd)

Table 1-6. Descriptions of Diseases for Which Therapeutic Apheresis Is Recommended* (Continued)

POLYCYTHEMIA VERA (PV) AND ERYTHROCYTOSIS

Condition	Procedure	Recommendation	Category
PV	Erythrocytapheresis	Grade 1B	I
Secondary erythrocytosis	Erythrocytapheresis	Grade 1C	III

Volume treated: volume of blood removed is based on the TBV, starting Hct, and desired postprocedure Hct

Replacement fluid: albumin

Frequency: as needed for symptomatic relief or to reach desired Hct (usually one)

Automated instruments allow the operator to choose a postprocedure Hct level and calculate the volume of blood removal necessary to attain the goal. A study found that using an exchange volume <15 mL/kg and inlet velocity <45 mL/minute, especially for patients >50 years old, may decrease adverse events. Saline boluses may be required during the procedure to reduce blood viscosity in the circuit and avoid pressure alarms.

In patients with PV, the goal is normalization of the Hct (ie, <45%). For secondary erythrocytosis, the goal is to relieve symptoms but retain a residual red cell mass that is optimal for tissue perfusion and oxygen delivery. A postprocedure Hct of 50% to 52% might be adequate for pulmonary hypoxia or high-oxygen-affinity hemoglobins, whereas Hct values of 55% to 60% might be optimal for patients with cyanotic congenital heart disease. A single procedure should be designed to achieve the desired postprocedure Hct.

POLYNEUROPATHY, ORGANOMEGALY, ENDOCRINOPATHY, M PROTEIN, AND SKIN CHANGES (POEMS)

Procedure	Recommendation	Category
TPE	Grade 1C	IV
Volume treated: 1-1.5 TPV	**Frequency:** mostly every other day (no standard)	
Replacement fluid: albumin		

Duration of treatment is variable in literature.

POSTTRANSFUSION PURPURA

Procedure	Recommendation	Category
TPE	Grade 2C	III
Volume treated: 1-1.5 TPV	**Frequency:** daily	
Replacement fluid: albumin, plasma		

Because of severe thrombocytopenia, the whole blood:AC ratio should be adjusted accordingly. Typically the replacement fluid is albumin to avoid further exposure to human platelet antigen (HPA)-1a. However, in bleeding patients, a plasma supplement can be given toward the end of procedure.

TPE can be discontinued when platelet count starts increasing (>20 × 10^9/L) and noncutaneous bleeding stops.

(cont'd)

Table 1-6. Descriptions of Diseases for Which Therapeutic Apheresis Is Recommended* (Continued)

PSORIASIS

Condition	Procedure	Recommendation	Category
Disseminated pustular	TPE	Grade 2 C	IV
	Adsorptive cytapheresis	Grade 2 C	III
	Lymphocytapheresis	Grade 2 C	III
	ECP	Grade 2 B	III

Volume treated—adsorption: 1500-2000 mL; **lymphocytapheresis:** 1500-5000 mL (1 TBV); **ECP:** 1000-3000 mL (method dependent)

Frequency—adsorption: once a week; **lymphocytapheresis:** once a week; **ECP:** once a week to twice a week

Replacement fluid—adsorption: NA; **lymphocytapheresis:** NA; **ECP:** NA

The granulocyte-monocyte adsorptive columns are not available in the United States.

Adsorptive columns and lymphocytapheresis are generally used for 5 weeks (total of five treatments). ECP has been used for different lengths of time (2-12 weeks) and hence needs to be adjusted based on the patient's presentation, as well as the objective of the treatment.

RED CELL ALLOIMMUNIZATION IN PREGNANCY

Condition	Procedure	Recommendation	Category
Before IUT availability	TPE	Grade 2C	III

Volume treated: 1-1.5 TPV   **Frequency**: three procedures per week

Replacement fluid: albumin

IUT = intrauterine transfusion.

TPE can safely be performed during pregnancy. Physiologically, blood and plasma volumes increase as the pregnancy progresses. In the second or third trimester, the patient should lay on her left side to avoid compression of the inferior vena cava by the gravid uterus. Hypotension should be avoided, as it may result in decreased perfusion to the fetus.

TPE should be considered early in pregnancy (from 7-20 weeks) and continued until IUT can safely be administered (about 20 weeks' gestation). Close monitoring of the fetus for signs of hydrops will aid in guiding treatment. One approach is to use TPE for the first week (three procedures) after the 12th week of pregnancy, followed by weekly IVIG (1 g/kg) until the 20th week.

(cont'd)

Table 1-6. Descriptions of Diseases for Which Therapeutic Apheresis Is Recommended* (Continued)

RENAL TRANSPLANTATION, ABO COMPATIBLE

Condition	Procedure	Recommendation	Category
Antibody-mediated rejection	TPE	Grade 1B	I
Desensitization, LD	TPE	Grade 1B	I
Desensitization, DD	TPE	Grade 2C	III

Volume treated: 1-1.5 TPV   **Frequency:** daily or every other day
Replacement fluid: albumin, plasma

LD = living donor; DD = deceased donor.

Patients should be started on immunosuppressive drugs before initiating TPE, to limit antibody resynthesis. For desensitization protocols, there appears to be a correlation between the number of TPEs needed preoperatively to obtain a negative crossmatch and the antibody titer.

For antibody-mediated rejection (AMR), some protocols use a set number of procedures, usually five or six, daily or every other day. Other protocols guide the number of treatments based on improvement in renal function and decrease in donor specific antibody titers. It is also undecided whether low-dose IVIG (100 mg/kg) should be used after every procedure or at the end of the series or not at all.

For desensitization protocols, TPE is performed daily or every other day per protocol until the crossmatch becomes negative. TPE is also performed postoperatively for a minimum of three procedures. Further treatment is determined by the risk of AMR, donor-specific antibody titers, or the occurrence of AMR.

88

RENAL TRANSPLANTATION, ABO INCOMPATIBLE (ABOI)

Condition	Procedure	Recommendation	Category
Desensitization, LD	TPE	Grade 1B	I
Humoral rejection	TPE	Grade 1B	II
A_2/A_2B into B, DD	TPE	Grade 1B	IV

Volume treated: 1-1.5 TPV   **Frequency**: daily or every other day

Replacement fluid: albumin, plasma

LD = living donor; DD = deceased donor.

The replacement fluid for TPE is albumin with or without use of plasma (plasma should be compatible with both the recipient and donor), depending on presence or absence of coagulopathy. In the immediate pretransplant setting, plasma or plasma/albumin is typically used.

The goal should be to reduce the antibody titer to less than a critical threshold before taking the patient to transplantation. It is important to note that this critical titer will need to be determined by each program embarking on this type of transplant, given that titer results can vary widely depending on titration method and technique. The number of TPE procedures required in most reports has depended on baseline IgG (not IgM) titer and the efficiency with which ABO antibodies are removed with TPE in the patient. Titers in the first 2 weeks afterward have a low positive predictive and high negative predictive value for antibody-mediated rejection (AMR) in the setting of ABOi renal transplantation. Most AMR episodes occur

(cont'd)

Table 1-6. Descriptions of Diseases for Which Therapeutic Apheresis Is Recommended* (Continued)

within the first 2 weeks following transplantation. Patients should be monitored closely for graft function before discontinuation of TPE. Several ABOi programs use protocol biopsies to monitor the allograft for histologic signs of rejection before discontinuation of TPE. Of note, c4d positivity is very common in ABOi transplant renal biopsies; however, this is not necessarily indicative of AMR unless accompanied by light microscopic changes suggestive of AMR.

SCLERODERMA (PROGRESSIVE SYSTEMIC SCLEROSIS)

Procedure	Recommendation	Category
TPE	Grade 2C	III
ECP	Grade 2A	III

Volume treated—ECP: MNC product of 200-270 mL; the two-process method collects and treats MNCs obtained from two-TBV processing; **TPE:** 1-1.5 TPV

Replacement fluid—ECP: NA; **TPE:** albumin

Frequency—ECP: Two procedures on consecutive days (one series) every 4 to 6 weeks for at least 6 to 9 months; TPE: one to three per week

The length of treatment with TPE varies widely. A course of six procedures over the course of 2 to 3 weeks should constitute a sufficient therapeutic trial. The treatment with ECP is longer, and likely at least a 6-month trial should be considered.

(cont'd)

91

Table 1-6. Descriptions of Diseases for Which Therapeutic Apheresis Is Recommended* (Continued)

SEPSIS WITH MULTIORGAN FAILURE

Procedure	Recommendation	Category
TPE	Grade 2B	III

Volume treated: 1-1.5 TPV **Frequency:** daily
Replacement fluid: plasma

Both centrifugal-based and filtration-based apheresis instruments have been used in the trials of TPE. Studies have also employed dialysis techniques combined with apheresis. Patients with or without severe coagulopathy are usually treated with plasma as a replacement fluid. Because these patients are severely ill with hypotension and cardiovascular instability, treatment should be performed in an appropriate setting, such as an ICU.

The above statements refer to reports of the use of TPE in the treatment of sepsis. In addition to TPE, a number of selective-removal columns have also been examined; polymyxin B and Matisse columns both bind endotoxin and have been shown to lower mortality or decrease ICU stay in RCTs, respectively. These columns were used to treat 1 to 1.5 blood volumes daily for 4 days. Neither of these devices has been approved for use in the United States.

One RCT limited treatment to one or two TPEs. Another RCT performed up to 14 TPEs. Case series have treated patients daily until improvement with different endpoints.

SICKLE CELL DISEASE, ACUTE

Condition	Procedure	Recommendation	Category
Acute stroke	RBC exchange	Grade 1C	I
Acute chest syndrome, severe	RBC exchange	Grade 1C	II
Priapism	RBC exchange	Grade 2C	III
Multiorgan failure	RBC exchange	Grade 2C	III
Splenic/hepatic sequestration; intrahepatic cholestasis	RBC exchange	Grade 2C	III

Volume treated: volume necessary to achieve target HbS level

Frequency: one procedure to achieve target HbS level

Replacement fluid: HbS-negative leukocyte-reduced RBCs, antigen-matched (if available) for at least C, E, and K

HbS = hemoglobin S.

93

Apheresis equipment calculates the replacement RBC volume to achieve the desired target HbS (FCR, the desired fraction of patient red cells remaining at the end of the procedure) and Hct levels. General guidelines to calculate replacement volume using the COBE Spectra (Terumo BCT, Lakewood, CO) are 1) end Hct at 30% ± 3% ($\leq$33-36% to avoid hyperviscosity), and 2) HbS of 30% (or HbS + HbC of 30%, etc). One can assume FCR at 25% to 40% in remotely transfused/never-transfused patients. In recently transfused patients, FCR can be calculated by dividing the desired HbS level by the preapheresis HbS level multiplied by 100. To maintain iso-

(cont'd)

Table 1-6. Descriptions of Diseases for Which Therapeutic Apheresis Is Recommended* (Continued)

volemia, primed saline is not diverted, and rinseback is omitted at the end of the run. In children and clinically unstable or severely anemic patients, 5% albumin may be used for priming.

For an acute situation, typically one procedure is necessary to achieve the desired HbS level (usually <30%) and end Hct (usually 30%).

SICKLE CELL DISEASE, NONACUTE

Condition	Procedure	Recommendation	Category
Stroke prophylaxis/iron over-load prevention	RBC exchange	Grade 1C	II
			III
Vaso-occlusive pain crisis	RBC exchange	Grade 2C	
Preoperative management	RBC exchange	Grade 2A	III

Volume treated: volume necessary to achieve target HbS level

Replacement fluid: HbS-negative leukocyte-reduced RBCs, antigen matched (if available) for at least C, E, and K

Frequency: as needed to maintain target HbS level

HbS = hemoglobin S.

Apheresis equipment calculates the replacement RBC volume to achieve the desired target HbS (FCR, the desired fraction of patient red cells remaining at the end of the procedure) and Hct levels. General guidelines to calculate replacement volume using the COBE Spectra (Terumo BCT, Lakewood, CO) are 1) end Hct at 30% ± 3% (≤33-36% to avoid hyperviscosity), and 2) HbS of 30% (or HbS + HbC of 30%, etc). One can assume FCR at 25% to 40% in remotely transfused/never-transfused patients. In recently transfused patients, FCR can be calculated by dividing the desired HbS level by the preapheresis HbS level multiplied by 100. To maintain iso-volemia, primed saline is not diverted, and rinseback is omitted at the end of the run. In children and clinically unstable or severely anemic patients, 5% albumin may be used for priming. Modification of RBC exchange using isovolemic hemodilution, which con-

(cont'd)

95

Table 1-6. Descriptions of Diseases for Which Therapeutic Apheresis Is Recommended* (Continued)

sists of RBC depletion with 0.9% NaCl replacement followed by standard RBC exchange, reduces replacement RBC volume and thus, potentially, donor exposure.

The duration and number of RBC exchanges depend on clinical indications; for example, one time for preoperative preparations, variable times for chronic pain, and lifelong exchange transfusion for stroke prevention, etc.

STIFF-PERSON SYNDROME

Procedure	Recommendation	Category
TPE	Grade 2C	III
Volume treated: 1-1.5 TPV	Frequency: every 1-3 days	
Replacement fluid: albumin		

TPE can effectively deplete antibodies of the IgG class when sufficient plasma volumes are exchanged in a brief period of time. If TPE is to be offered to a patient with stiff-person syndrome, the patient should be made aware of the paucity of clinical data to support its use and also of the availability of IVIG as an alternative. If IVIG is not available, then it may be reasonable to proceed with TPE. TPE may be considered also if the patient does not respond to conventional therapy. TPE should be used as an adjunct with standard pharmacologic therapy.

A series of four to five plasma exchanges of 1 to 1.5 plasma volumes performed over 8 to 14 days should effectively deplete IgG. Repeat series of plasma exchange can be employed empirically if there is an objective clinical improvement that is followed by a relapse of symptoms.

(cont'd)

Table 1-6. Descriptions of Diseases for Which Therapeutic Apheresis Is Recommended* (Continued)

SUDDEN SENSORINEURAL HEARING LOSS

Procedure	Recommendation	Category
LDL apheresis	Grade 2A	III
Rheopheresis	Grade 2A	III
TPE	Grade 2C	III

Volume treated—LDL apheresis: 3 L; **rheopheresis:** 1 TPV; **TPE:** 1 TPV

Replacement fluid—LDL apheresis: NA; **rheopheresis:** NA; **TPE:** albumin

Frequency—LDL apheresis: one to two; **rheopheresis:** one to two; **TPE:** three every other day

Patients with LDL cholesterol or fibrinogen elevations respond to apheresis treatment more rapidly and with greater improvement. Specific trigger levels have not, however, been suggested. Longer time between symptom onset and treatment is associated with poorer hearing recovery.

For HELP and rheopheresis, one to two procedures were performed on consecutive days, depending on response as determined by standard audiometry. In the TPE case series, treatment was repeated if the patient's hearing deteriorated after initial improvement.

SYSTEMIC LUPUS ERYTHEMATOSUS (SLE)

Condition	Procedure	Recommendation	Category
Severe	TPE	Grade 2C	II
Nephritis	TPE	Grade 1B	IV

Volume treated: 1-1.5 TPV

Frequency—lupus cerebritis or SLE with DAH: daily or every other day; **SLE (other):** one to three times per week

Replacement fluid: albumin, plasma

Typically a course of three to six TPEs is sufficient to see response in the patients with lupus cerebritis or DAH. Prolonged treatments have been reported, but their efficacy and rationale is questionable.

99

(cont'd)

Table 1-6. Descriptions of Diseases for Which Therapeutic Apheresis Is Recommended* (Continued)

THROMBOCYTOSIS

Condition	Procedure	Recommendation	Category
Symptomatic	Thrombocytapheresis	Grade 2C	II
Prophylactic or secondary	Thrombocytapheresis	Grade 2C	III

Volume treated: 1.5 to 2 TBV **Frequency:** daily or as indicated to reach/maintain goal
Replacement fluid: saline

Each procedure lowers the platelet count by 30% to 60%. A central venous catheter may be required for multiple treatments or long-term therapy. The ratio of whole blood:anticoagulant should be 1:6-12, and heparin should be avoided to prevent ex-vivo platelet clumping. Methods of thrombocytapheresis typically differ from donor plateletapheresis; thus, manufacturers' recommendations as well as published reports should be carefully considered before initiation of the procedure.

With acute thromboembolism or hemorrhage, the goal is normalization of the platelet count and maintenance of a normal count until cytoreductive therapy takes effect. The goal for prophylaxis of high-risk patients who are pregnant, who are undergoing surgery, or who have had splenectomy should be determined on a case-by-case basis (eg, considering the patient's history of thrombosis or bleeding at a specific platelet count). Without an informative clinical history, a platelet count of 600×10^9/L or less may be sufficient.

THROMBOTIC MICROANGIOPATHY (TMA), DRUG ASSOCIATED

Condition	Procedure	Recommendation	Category
Ticlopidine	TPE	Grade 2B	I
Clopidogrel	TPE	Grade 1B	III
Cyclosporine/tacrolimus	TPE	Grade 2C	III
Gemcitabine	TPE	Grade 2C	IV
Quinine	TPE	Grade 2C	IV

Volume treated: 1-1.5 TPV   **Frequency:** daily or every other day

Replacement fluid: plasma, plasma cryoprecipitate removed

The specific TPE replacement fluid strategy and frequency are not described in the majority of published case reports. The pattern of response of platelet count, hematologic and laboratory parameters, and clinical signs may be variable and incomplete compared to patients undergoing TPE for idiopathic TTP. Otherwise, similar procedural considerations apply as for TPE used in TTP.

TPE for drug-associated TMA is usually performed daily until recovery of hematologic parameters, and then either discontinued or tapered off, similar to treatment for idiopathic TTP. The therapeutic endpoint may be difficult to determine or attain because of confounding morbidity from underlying disease or other factors not yet recognized. The durability of response and frequency of relapse are undefined. Reexposure to the associated drug should be avoided.

(cont'd)

Table 1-6. Descriptions of Diseases for Which Therapeutic Apheresis Is Recommended* (Continued)

THROMBOTIC MICROANGIOPATHY, HEMATOPOIETIC STEM CELL TRANSPLANT ASSOCIATED (TA-TMA)

Condition	Procedure	Recommendation	Category
Refractory	TPE	Grade 2C	III

Volume treated: 1-1.5 TPV

Frequency: daily, or as indicated for chronic management

Replacement fluid: plasma, plasma cryoprecipitate removed

TPE for patients with TA-TMA is often complicated by thrombocytopenia, anemia, and the comorbidities related to graft-vs-host disease and infections, including bleeding and hypotension. Therefore, the pattern of platelet and LDH responses may be variable and incomplete compared to patients undergoing TPE for idiopathic TTP. Otherwise, similar procedural considerations apply as for TPE used in TTP.

TPE for TA-TMA is usually performed daily until a response occurs, and then either discontinued or tapered off, similar to treatment for idiopathic TTP. The therapeutic endpoint may be difficult to determine because the platelet count and LDH levels could be affected by incomplete engraftment and posttransplant complications. Because microangiopathic hemolytic anemia may be caused by other disorders and drugs after transplantation, isolated persistence of schistocytes on the peripheral blood smear, without other clinical manifestations of TMA, may not preclude discontinuation of treatment.

THROMBOTIC THROMBOCYTOPENIC PURPURA (TTP)

Procedure	Recommendation	Category
TPE	Grade 1A	I

Volume treated: 1-1.5 TPV **Frequency:** daily

Replacement fluid: plasma, plasma cryoprecipitate removed

Transfusion of RBCs, when medically necessary, may be given emergently during TPE. Clinical response with clearing of mental status usually precedes recovery of platelet count and normalization of LDH. The median number of TPE procedures to establish hematologic recovery is 7 to 8 daily treatments. The pattern of platelet response is variable, and platelet count may fluctuate during treatment. Allergic reactions and citrate reactions are more frequent as a result of the large volumes of plasma required. Because plasma has citrate as an anticoagulant, ACD-A can be used in a higher ratio to minimize citrate reactions, especially with moderate to severe thrombocytopenia. Fibrinogen levels may decrease following serial TPE procedures with plasma cryoprecipitate removed used as replacement. In patients with severe allergic reactions to plasma proteins or a limited supply of ABO-compatible plasma, 5% albumin may be substituted for the initial portion (up to 50%) of replacement. Albumin alone, however, has never been shown efficacy.

TPE is generally performed daily until the platelet count is above 150×10^9/L and LDH is near normal for 2 to 3 consecutive days. The role of tapering TPE over a longer duration has not been studied prospectively, but tapering is used frequently. Persistence of schistocytes alone on peripheral blood smear, in the absence of other clinical features of TTP, does not preclude discontinuation of treatment.

(cont'd)

Table 1-6. Descriptions of Diseases for Which Therapeutic Apheresis Is Recommended* (Continued)

THYROID STORM

Procedure	Recommendation	Category
TPE	Grade 2C	III
Volume treated: 1-1.5 TPV	**Frequency:** daily or every 2 to 3 days	
Replacement fluid: plasma, albumin		

Plasma as replacement fluid has the advantage of increasing the concentration of thyroglobulin to bind free thyroid hormone. TPE should be continued until clinical improvement is noted.

TOXIC EPIDERMAL NECROLYSIS (TEN)

Condition	Procedure	Recommendation	Category
Refractory	TPE	Grade 2B	III

Volume treated: 1-1.5 PV **Frequency:** daily or every other day

Replacement fluid: plasma, albumin

Although most reports have used TPE to treat refractory TEN, some groups from Japan have also used double-filtration plasmapheresis, which is not available in the United States.

The number of TPE treatments varies considerably, from one to more than five procedures, and discontinuation has been guided by clinical improvement (most frequently skin healing and reepithelialization).

(cont'd)

105

Table 1-6. Descriptions of Diseases for Which Therapeutic Apheresis Is Recommended* (Continued)

VOLTAGE-GATED POTASSIUM CHANNEL (VGKC) ANTIBODY-RELATED DISEASES

Procedure	Recommendation	Category
TPE	Grade 1C	II
Volume treated: 1-1.5 TPV	**Frequency:** every other day	
Replacement fluid: albumin		

Some investigators suggest using 50-mL/kg plasma exchange; however, there are no strong data to support this volume. The patients who present with seizures should be adequately protected against self-injury if seizure activity occurs during performance of the apheresis procedure. Some of the patients, because of their memory loss and other neuropsychiatric symptoms, might not be able to provide good histories, so involvement of family members in evaluation of the response to treatment in addition to formal evaluation can be helpful. These patients may also exhibit emotional and physical outbursts; hence, additional precautions might be necessary for the staff until the patient reaction to the environment and treatment is established.

Five to seven TPE procedures over 7 to 14 days are recommended. The assessment of VGKC antibody levels is suggested after the series of treatments to evaluate the response. It has been shown that the level of antibody correlates with severity of the symptoms. The response to the treatment might be delayed, so additional treatments beyond 7 are not generally recommended.

WILSON DISEASE

Condition	Procedure	Recommendation	Category
Fulminant	TPE	Grade 1C	I

Volume treated: 1-1.5 TPV

Frequency: daily or every other day

Replacement fluid: plasma, albumin

Replacement of the patient's plasma with Fresh Frozen Plasma provides additional coagulation factors and rapidly corrects coagulopathy. A combination of plasma and albumin is also possible. Use of albumin alone will worsen coagulopathy.

The reduction in serum copper in most case reports had been achieved rapidly and maintained after the first two treatments. However, daily TPE can be beneficial if the patient has acute hepatic failure with coagulopathy until liver transplantation is performed. The specific laboratory tests for the disease (eg, serum copper, 24-hour urinary copper excretion) are not routine testing and thus are not helpful to guide effectiveness and the frequency of the treatment. In most cases, judgment might be based on clinical parameters and routine testing (ie, improved encephalopathy, controlled hemolysis, decrease in liver function test abnormalities, etc).

*Modified from Schwartz J, Winters JL, Padmanabhan A, et al. Guidelines on the use of therapeutic apheresis in clinical practice—Evidence-based approach from the Apheresis Applications Committee of the American Society for Apheresis. The Sixth Special Issue. J Clin Apheresis 2013;28: 145-284.

(cont'd)

Table 1-6. Descriptions of Diseases for Which Therapeutic Apheresis Is Recommended* (Continued)

Abbreviations: ACD-A = acid-citrate-dextrose, formula A; ACE = angiotensin-converting enzyme; apoB = apolipoprotein B; CNS = central nervous system; DAH = diffuse alveolar hemorrhage; ECP = extracorporeal photopheresis; ELISA = enzyme-linked immunosorbent assay; FDA = Food and Drug Administration; GI = gastrointestinal; Hct = hematocrit; HELP = heparin extracorporeal LDL precipitation; HIPA = heparin-induced platelet activation test; HPC = hematopoietic progenitor cell; IA = immunoabsorption; ICU = intensive care unit; IVIG = intravenous immunoglobulin; LDH = lactate dehydrogenase; LDL = low-density lipoprotein; Lp(a) = lipoprotein (a); MNC = mononuclear cell; NA = not applicable; NYHA = New York Heart Association; RBC = red blood cell; RCT = randomized controlled trial; RPGN = rapidly progressive glomerulonephritis; TBV = total blood volume; TPE = therapeutic plasma exchange; TPV = total plasma volume; TTP = thrombotic thrombocytopenic purpura; WBC = white blood cell.

Table 1-7. Considerations When Evaluating a New Patient for Therapeutic Apheresis*

General	Description
Rationale[†]	Based on the established/presumptive diagnosis and history of present illness, the discussion could include the rationale for the procedure, a brief account of the results of published studies, and patient-specific risks from the procedure
Impact	The effect of therapeutic apheresis on comorbidities and medications (and vice versa) should be considered
Technical issues[†]	The technical aspects of therapeutic apheresis, such as type of anticoagulant, replacement solution, vascular access, and volume of whole blood processed (eg, number of plasma volumes exchanged), should be addressed
Therapeutic plan[†]	Total number and/or frequency of therapeutic apheresis procedures should be addressed

(cont'd)

109

Table 1-7. Considerations When Evaluating a New Patient for Therapeutic Apheresis*
(Continued)

General	Description
Clinical and/or laboratory endpoints[†]	The clinical and/or laboratory parameters should be established to monitor effectiveness of the treatment.
	The criteria for discontinuation of therapeutic apheresis should be discussed whenever appropriate
Timing and location	The acceptable timing of initiation of therapeutic apheresis should be considered on the basis of clinical considerations (eg, medical emergency, urgent, routine etc). The location where the therapeutic apheresis will take place should be also addressed (eg, intensive care unit, medical ward, operating room, outpatient setting). If timing appropriate to the clinical condition and urgency level cannot be met, a transfer to a different facility should be considered according to the clinical status of the patient.

The above issues should be considered in addition to a routine note addressing patient's history, review of systems, and physical examination.

*Modified from Schwartz J, Winters JL, Padmanabhan A, et al. Guidelines on the use of therapeutic apheresis in clinical practice—Evidence-based approach from the Apheresis Applications Committee of the American Society for Apheresis. The Sixth Special Issue. J Clin Apheresis 2013;28:145-284.

[†]The American Society for Apheresis Fact Sheet for each disease could be helpful in addressing these issues.

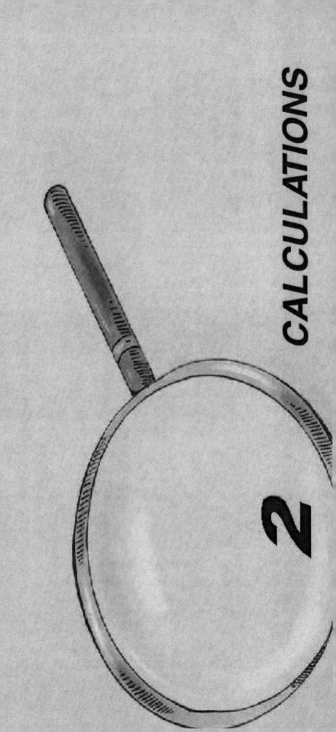

2

CALCULATIONS

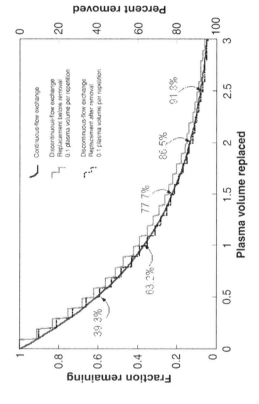

Figure 2-1. The relationship between the volume of plasma exchange and the patient's remaining original plasma. Used with permission from Brecher ME, ed. Technical manual. 15th ed. Bethesda, MD: AABB, 2005:149.

Table 2-1. Alteration in Blood Constituents by a Single-Plasma-Volume Exchange*†

Constituent	Percent Decrease from Baseline	Percent Recovery 48 Hours after Plasma Exchange
Clotting factors	25–50	80–100
Fibrinogen	63	65
Immunoglobulins	63	~45
Paraproteins	30–60	Variable
Liver enzymes	55–60	100
Bilirubin	45	100
C3	63	60–100
Platelets	25–30	75–100

*Used with permission from Weinstein R. Basic principles of therapeutic blood exchange. In: McLeod BC, Weinstein R, Winters JL, Szczepiorkowski ZM, eds. Apheresis: Principles and practice. 3rd ed. Bethesda, MD: AABB Press, 2010:277.

†Replacement fluid consisting of 4%-5% albumin in 0.9% sodium chloride.

113

Table 2-2. Total Blood Volume*

Age Group	Approximate Blood Volume (mL/kg)
Premature infant, at birth	90-105
Term newborn infant	80-90
Children (>3 months)	70-75
Adolescents and adults	
Male	70
Female	65

*Used with permission from Winters JL, King K, eds. Therapeutic apheresis: A physician's handbook. 4th ed. Bethesda, MD: AABB, 2013.

Table 2-3. Calculation of Total Blood Volume*

Gilcher's Rule of Fives

Patient	Blood Volume (mL/kg of Body Weight)			
	Fat	Thin	Normal	Muscular
Male	60	65	70	75
Female	55	60	65	70

Nadler's Formula

Patient	Total Blood Volume (mL)
Male	$(0.006012 \times H^3)/(14.6 \times W) + 604$
Female	$(0.005835 \times H^3)/(15 \times W) + 183$

*Used with permission from Chhibber V, King KE. Management of the therapeutic apheresis patient. In: McLeod BC, Weinstein R, Winters JL, Szczepiorkowski ZM, eds. Apheresis: Principles and practice. 2nd ed. Bethesda, MD: AABB Press, 2011:232.
H = height in inches; W = weight in pounds.

Table 2-4. Estimated Red Cell Volume in Liters for Different Body Weights, Blood Volumes, and Hematocrits

Weight (in kg)	Blood Volume (in liters)*	Hematocrit (%)								
		15	20	25	30	35	40	45	50
10	0.7	0.1	0.1	0.2	0.2	0.2	0.3	0.3	0.4
15	1.1	0.2	0.2	0.3	0.3	0.4	0.4	0.5	0.5
20	1.4	0.2	0.3	0.4	0.4	0.5	0.6	0.6	0.7
25	1.8	0.3	0.4	0.4	0.5	0.6	0.7	0.8	0.9
30	2.1	0.3	0.4	0.5	0.6	0.7	0.8	0.9	1.1
35	2.5	0.4	0.5	0.6	0.7	0.9	1.0	1.1	1.2
40	2.8	0.4	0.6	0.7	0.8	1.0	1.1	1.3	1.4
45	3.2	0.5	0.6	0.8	0.9	1.1	1.3	1.4	1.6
50	3.5	0.5	0.7	0.9	1.1	1.2	1.4	1.6	1.8
55	3.9	0.6	0.8	1.0	1.2	1.3	1.5	1.7	1.9
60	4.2	0.6	0.8	1.1	1.3	1.5	1.7	1.9	2.1
65	4.6	0.7	0.9	1.1	1.4	1.6	1.8	2.0	2.3
70	4.9	0.7	1.0	1.2	1.5	1.7	2.0	2.2	2.5
75	5.3	0.8	1.1	1.3	1.6	1.8	2.1	2.4	2.6

80	5.6	0.8	1.1	1.4	1.7	2.0	2.2	2.5	2.8
85	6.0	0.9	1.2	1.5	1.8	2.1	2.4	2.7	3.0
90	6.3	0.9	1.3	1.6	1.9	2.2	2.5	2.8	3.2
95	6.7	1.0	1.3	1.7	2.0	2.3	2.7	3.0	3.3
100	7.0	1.1	1.4	1.8	2.1	2.5	2.8	3.2	3.5
105	7.4	1.1	1.5	1.8	2.2	2.6	2.9	3.3	3.7
110	7.7	1.2	1.5	1.9	2.3	2.7	3.1	3.5	3.9
115	8.1	1.2	1.6	2.0	2.4	2.8	3.2	3.6	4.0
120	8.4	1.3	1.7	2.1	2.5	2.9	3.4	3.8	4.2
125	8.8	1.3	1.8	2.2	2.6	3.1	3.5	3.9	4.4
130	9.1	1.4	1.8	2.3	2.7	3.2	3.6	4.1	4.6
135	9.5	1.4	1.9	2.4	2.8	3.3	3.8	4.3	4.7
140	9.8	1.5	2.0	2.5	2.9	3.4	3.9	4.4	4.9
145	10.2	1.5	2.0	2.5	3.0	3.6	4.1	4.6	5.1
150	10.5	1.6	2.1	2.6	3.2	3.7	4.2	4.7	5.3

*Based on 70 mL/kg.

117

Table 2-5. Estimated Plasma Volume in Liters for Different Body Weights, Blood Volumes, and Hematocrits

Weight (in kg)	Blood Volume (in liters)*	Hematocrit							
		15	20	25	30	35	40	45	50
10	0.7	0.6	0.6	0.5	0.5	0.5	0.4	0.4	0.4
15	1.1	0.9	0.8	0.8	0.7	0.7	0.6	0.6	0.5
20	1.4	1.2	1.1	1.1	1.0	0.9	0.8	0.8	0.7
25	1.8	1.5	1.4	1.3	1.2	1.1	1.1	1.0	0.9
30	2.1	1.8	1.7	1.6	1.5	1.4	1.3	1.2	1.1
35	2.5	2.1	2.0	1.8	1.7	1.6	1.5	1.3	1.2
40	2.8	2.4	2.2	2.1	2.0	1.8	1.7	1.5	1.4
45	3.2	2.7	2.5	2.4	2.2	2.0	1.9	1.7	1.6
50	3.5	3.0	2.8	2.6	2.5	2.3	2.1	1.9	1.8
55	3.9	3.3	3.1	2.9	2.7	2.5	2.3	2.1	1.9
60	4.2	3.6	3.4	3.2	2.9	2.7	2.5	2.3	2.1
65	4.6	3.9	3.6	3.4	3.2	3.0	2.7	2.5	2.3
70	4.9	4.2	3.9	3.7	3.4	3.2	2.9	2.7	2.5
75	5.3	4.5	4.2	3.9	3.7	3.4	3.2	2.9	2.6

80	5.6	4.8	4.5	4.2	3.9	3.6	3.4	3.1	2.8
85	6.0	5.1	4.8	4.5	4.2	3.9	3.6	3.3	3.0
90	6.3	5.4	5.0	4.7	4.4	4.1	3.8	3.5	3.2
95	6.7	5.7	5.3	5.0	4.7	4.3	4.0	3.7	3.3
100	7.0	6.0	5.6	5.3	4.9	4.6	4.2	3.9	3.5
105	7.4	6.2	5.9	5.5	5.1	4.8	4.4	4.0	3.7
110	7.7	6.5	6.2	5.8	5.4	5.0	4.6	4.2	3.9
115	8.1	6.8	6.4	6.0	5.6	5.2	4.8	4.4	4.0
120	8.4	7.1	6.7	6.3	5.9	5.5	5.0	4.6	4.2
125	8.8	7.4	7.0	6.6	6.1	5.7	5.3	4.8	4.4
130	9.1	7.7	7.3	6.8	6.4	5.9	5.5	5.0	4.6
135	9.5	8.0	7.6	7.1	6.6	6.1	5.7	5.2	4.7
140	9.8	8.3	7.8	7.4	6.9	6.4	5.9	5.4	4.9
145	10.2	8.6	8.1	7.6	7.1	6.6	6.1	5.6	5.1
150	10.5	8.9	8.4	7.9	7.4	6.8	6.3	5.8	5.3

*Based on 70 mL/kg.

119

Table 2-6. Sample Calculations and Predictions*

Formula	Calculation	Net Volume
Calculations		
Total blood volume (TBV) = 70 mL/kg × wt	(70 mL/kg) × (10 kg)	700 mL
Red cell volume (RV) = Hct × TBV	(0.3) × (700 mL)	210 mL
Plasma volume (PV) = (1 − Hct) × TBV	(1 − 0.3) × (700 mL)	490 mL
Predictions with Standard Procedure†		
A. Extracorporeal blood volume (EBV)		
Intraprocedure volume loss		−150 mL
Device- and procedure-specific		
Percentage EBV	$\dfrac{150 \text{ mL}}{700 \text{ mL}} \times 100$	21%
(EBV ÷ TBV) × 100		

B. Extracorporeal RV (ERV)

ERV loss $\quad\quad\quad\quad\quad\quad$ 68 mL + (36 mL × 0.3) $\quad\quad\quad\quad$ −79 mL

$\quad$ Device- and procedure-specific

$\quad\quad$ COBE Spectra = 68 mL

$\quad\quad$ COBE SpectraTherm blood warmer ECV = 36 mL

Percentage ERV $\quad\quad\quad\quad\quad\quad \dfrac{79\ mL}{210\ mL} \times 100 \quad\quad\quad\quad$ 38%

$\quad$ (ERV ÷ RV) × 100 = %ERV

Intraprocedure Hct $\quad\quad\quad\quad \dfrac{(210-79)\ mL}{700\ mL} \times 100 \quad\quad\quad\quad$ 19%

$\quad \dfrac{(RV - ERV)}{TBV} \times 100 = IH$

---

*Used with permission from Eder AF, Kim HC. Pediatric therapeutic apheresis. In: Herman JH, Manno CS, eds. Pediatric transfusion therapy. Bethesda, MD: AABB Press, 2002:471-508.

†Plasmapheresis, COBE Spectra, dual-needle operation, diverting prime saline ERV equals COBE Spectra red cell requirement to establish the plasma–red cell interface within the channel (68 mL) in addition to the red cells in the blood warmer [ECV × Hct of blood in warmer]. Examples given are for a child with a body wt of 10 kg and a Hct of 30%. Consequently, the standard procedure should be modified to include blood prime and to ensure fluid and red cell balance throughout the procedure.

ECV = extracorporeal volume; Hct = hematocrit; IH = intraoperative hemodilution; wt = weight.

Table 2-7. Intravascular Volume and Red Cell Shifts*†

| | Net Intravascular Volume Shift (mL) | | Net Red Cell Volume Shift (mL)‡ | |
	Intraprocedure	Postprocedure	Intraprocedure	Postprocedure
Plasma exchange	–150	+195	–68	–15
Erythrocytapheresis	–100	+245	–68	–16
Leukocytapheresis, version 4.7	–150 + AC – white cells	+263 + AC – white cells	–114 – [red cell content in collected white cells]	–24 – [red cell content in collected white cells]
Leukocytapheresis, version 6.0	–150 + AC – white cells	+185 + AC – white cells	–66 – [red cell content in white cells]§	–9 – [red cell content in white cells]‡

*Adapted with permission from Eder AF, Kim HC. Pediatric therapeutic apheresis. In: Herman JH, Manno CS, eds. Pediatric transfusion therapy. Bethesda, MD: AABB Press, 2002:471-508.
†Using the COBE Spectra (CaridianBCT, Lakewood, CO) dual-needle operation, standard procedure (divert saline prime, perform rinseback).
‡Volume of blood warmer or other device added to the extracorporeal circuit is not included.
§Average red cell content (volume) in white cells collected = volume of white cells collected x hematocrit of white cell product/100.
AC = anticoagulant volume.

122

Table 2-8. Sample Calculations for Volume Shifts during Leukapheresis*†

Intravascular Volume Shifts	Formula and Calculation
Postprocedure volume loss (Table 2-7)	185 mL + anticoagulant – white cells: 185 mL + 460 mL – 1193 mL = –548 mL
% TBV	–548 mL ÷ 2030 mL = –27%
Red Cell Balance	
Total red cell volume	TBV × hematocrit: 2030 mL (0.26) = 528 mL
Intraprocedure red cell loss (maximum)	From Table 2-7: –66 mL – [red cell content in white cells] = –66 mL – [volume of white cells collected × hematocrit of white cell product/100] = –66 mL – [1193 mL × 0.07] = –150 mL

(cont'd)

Table 2-8. Sample Calculations for Volume Shifts during Leukapheresis*† (Continued)

Intravascular Volume Shifts	Formula and Calculation
Predicted intraprocedure hematocrit nadir of patient with isovolemic procedure	[528 mL – 150 mL]/2030 × 100% = 19%
Postprocedure red cell loss (after rinseback)	From Table 2-7: –9 mL – [red cell content of white cells] = –9 mL – [volume of white cells collected hematocrit of white cell product/100] = –9 mL – [1193 mL × 0.07] = –93 mL
Predicted postprocedure hematocrit of patient with isovolemic procedure	[528 mL – 93 mL]/2030 × 100% = 21%

*Used with permission from Winters JL, Gottschall JL, eds. Therapeutic apheresis: A physician's handbook. 3rd ed. Bethesda, MD, AABB, 2011:207.

†Calculations are for a 9-year-old child with T-cell acute lymphoblastic leukemia and who presented with an altered level of consciousness, a white cell count of 793,000/µL (90% blasts), and a hematocrit of 26%. For three blood volumes (6090 mL) processed on the COBE Spectra (CaridianBCT) with version 6.0 software, the predicted final volume collected with 1193 mL (hematocrit of collected product, 7%), when 460 mL anticoagulant was used.

TBV = total blood volume.

124

Table 2-9. Calculations for Volume Exchange in Manual Apheresis/Hemodilution

For isovolemic hemodilution, the following equation indicates the volume that must be exchanged (or lost) to achieve a final decrease in an analyte of interest (which could be circulating plasma protein or hematocrit) held exclusively in the intravascular space:

$$V_L = EBV \times \ln (A_0/A_F)$$

where A_0 = analyte concentration at time zero, A_F = analyte concentration at time final, V_L = volume loss, and EBV = estimated blood volume.

Although a manual push/pull technique is not a continuous process, if the volumes exchanged in each cycle are small compared to the total volume, this equation will approximate the actual answer.

For example, given a polycythemic child (35 kg, estimated blood volume = 2500 mL) for whom one is asked to reduce the hematocrit from 60% to 48% using 5% albumin as replacement, if a push/pull procedure is used (20 mL at a time), the total volume to withdraw and replace would be as follows:

$$2500 \times \ln (60/48) = 558 \text{ mL}$$

This would equal approximately 28 push/pull cycles (558/20).

Adapted with permission from Brecher ME, Hay SN. Collected questions and answers. 9th ed. Bethesda, MD: AABB, 2008:6.

Table 2-10. Mean Volumes in Liters to Process (Target Dose = 5×10^6/kg) for Different CD34 Concentrations

Weight (in kg)	5	7	10	15	20	25	50	75	100	125	150	175	200
							CD34/μL						
10	36.2	26.7	19.2	13.0	9.9	8.0	4.0	2.7	2.0	1.6	1.4	1.2	1.0
15	54.3	40.1	28.8	19.6	14.8	11.9	6.0	4.0	3.0	2.4	2.0	1.7	1.5
20	72.3	53.4	38.4	26.1	19.8	15.9	8.1	5.4	4.1	3.2	2.7	2.3	2.0
25	90.4	66.8	47.9	32.6	24.7	19.9	10.1	6.7	5.1	4.1	3.4	2.9	2.5
30	108.5	80.1	57.5	39.1	29.7	23.9	12.1	8.1	6.1	4.9	4.1	3.5	3.1
35	126.6	93.5	67.1	45.7	34.6	27.9	14.1	9.4	7.1	5.7	4.7	4.1	3.6
40	144.7	106.8	76.7	52.2	39.5	31.8	16.1	10.8	8.1	6.5	5.4	4.6	4.1
45	162.8	120.2	86.3	58.7	44.5	35.8	18.1	12.1	9.1	7.3	6.1	5.2	4.6
50	180.8	133.5	95.9	65.2	49.4	39.8	20.2	13.5	10.1	8.1	6.8	5.8	5.1
55	198.9	146.9	105.5	71.8	54.4	43.8	22.2	14.8	11.2	8.9	7.5	6.4	5.6
60	217.0	160.2	115.1	78.3	59.3	47.8	24.2	16.2	12.2	9.7	8.1	7.0	6.1
65	235.1	173.6	124.7	84.8	64.3	51.7	26.2	17.5	13.2	10.6	8.8	7.6	6.6
70	253.2	186.9	134.2	91.3	69.2	55.7	28.2	18.9	14.2	11.4	9.5	8.1	7.1

75	271.3	200.3	143.8	97.9	74.2	59.7	30.2	20.2	15.2	12.2	10.2	8.7	7.6
80	289.3	213.6	153.4	104.4	79.1	63.7	32.2	21.6	16.2	13.0	10.8	9.3	8.1
85	307.4	227.0	163.0	110.9	84.0	67.7	34.3	22.9	17.2	13.8	11.5	9.9	8.6
90	325.5	240.3	172.6	117.4	89.0	71.6	36.3	24.3	18.3	14.6	12.2	10.5	9.2
95	343.6	253.7	182.2	124.0	93.9	75.6	38.3	25.6	19.3	15.4	12.9	11.0	9.7
100	361.7	267.0	191.8	130.5	98.9	79.6	40.3	27.0	20.3	16.2	13.5	11.6	10.2
105	379.8	280.4	201.4	137.0	103.8	83.6	42.3	28.3	21.3	17.1	14.2	12.2	10.7
110	397.8	293.7	210.9	143.5	108.8	87.6	44.3	29.7	22.3	17.9	14.9	12.8	11.2
115	415.9	307.1	220.5	150.0	113.7	91.5	46.3	31.0	23.3	18.7	15.6	13.4	11.7
120	434.0	320.4	230.1	156.6	118.6	95.5	48.4	32.4	24.3	19.5	16.3	13.9	12.2
125	452.1	333.8	239.7	163.1	123.6	99.5	50.4	33.7	25.4	20.3	16.9	14.5	12.7
130	470.2	347.1	249.3	169.6	128.5	103.5	52.4	35.1	26.4	21.1	17.6	15.1	13.2
135	488.3	360.5	258.9	176.1	133.5	107.5	54.4	36.4	27.4	21.9	18.3	15.7	13.7
140	506.3	373.9	268.5	182.7	138.4	111.4	56.4	37.8	28.4	22.7	19.0	16.3	14.2
145	524.4	387.2	278.1	189.2	143.4	115.4	58.4	39.1	29.4	23.6	19.6	16.9	14.8
150	542.5	400.6	287.7	195.7	148.3	119.4	60.5	40.5	30.4	24.4	20.3	17.4	15.3

Table 2-11. Mean Volumes in Liters to Process (Target Dose = 6×10^6/kg) for Different CD34 Concentrations

Weight (in kg)	CD34/µL												
	5	7	10	15	20	25	50	75	100	125	150	175	200
10	43.4	32.0	23.0	15.7	11.9	9.6	4.8	3.2	2.4	1.9	1.6	1.4	1.2
15	65.1	48.1	34.5	23.5	17.8	14.3	7.3	4.9	3.7	2.9	2.4	2.1	1.8
20	86.8	64.1	46.0	31.3	23.7	19.1	9.7	6.5	4.9	3.9	3.3	2.8	2.4
25	108.5	80.1	57.5	39.1	29.7	23.9	12.1	8.1	6.1	4.9	4.1	3.5	3.1
30	130.2	96.1	69.0	47.0	35.6	28.7	14.5	9.7	7.3	5.8	4.9	4.2	3.7
35	151.9	112.2	80.5	54.8	41.5	33.4	16.9	11.3	8.5	6.8	5.7	4.9	4.3
40	173.6	128.2	92.0	62.6	47.5	38.2	19.3	13.0	9.7	7.8	6.5	5.6	4.9
45	195.3	144.2	103.6	70.5	53.4	43.0	21.8	14.6	11.0	8.8	7.3	6.3	5.5
50	217.0	160.2	115.1	78.3	59.3	47.8	24.2	16.2	12.2	9.7	8.1	7.0	6.1
55	238.7	176.2	126.6	86.1	65.3	52.5	26.6	17.8	13.4	10.7	8.9	7.7	6.7
60	260.4	192.3	138.1	93.9	71.2	57.3	29.0	19.4	14.6	11.7	9.8	8.4	7.3
65	282.1	208.3	149.6	101.8	77.1	62.1	31.4	21.0	15.8	12.7	10.6	9.1	7.9
70	303.8	224.3	161.1	109.6	83.1	66.9	33.9	22.7	17.0	13.6	11.4	9.8	8.5
75	325.5	240.3	172.6	117.4	89.0	71.6	36.3	24.3	18.3	14.6	12.2	10.5	9.2

80	347.2	256.4	184.1	125.3	94.9	76.4	38.7	25.9	19.5	15.6	13.0	11.2	9.8
85	368.9	272.4	195.6	133.1	100.9	81.2	41.1	27.5	20.7	16.6	13.8	11.9	10.4
90	390.6	288.4	207.1	140.9	106.8	86.0	43.5	29.1	21.9	17.5	14.6	12.6	11.0
95	412.3	304.4	218.6	148.7	112.7	90.7	45.9	30.8	23.1	18.5	15.4	13.2	11.6
100	434.0	320.4	230.1	156.6	118.6	5.5	48.4	32.4	24.3	19.5	16.3	13.9	12.2
105	455.7	336.5	241.6	164.4	124.6	100.3	50.8	34.0	25.6	20.5	17.1	14.6	12.8
110	477.4	352.5	253.1	172.2	130.5	105.1	53.2	35.6	26.8	21.4	17.9	15.3	13.4
115	499.1	368.5	264.6	180.1	136.4	109.8	55.6	37.2	28.0	22.4	18.7	16.0	14.0
120	520.8	384.5	276.1	187.9	142.4	114.6	58.0	38.9	29.2	23.4	19.5	16.7	14.6
125	542.5	400.6	287.7	195.7	148.3	119.4	60.5	40.5	30.4	24.4	20.3	17.4	15.3
130	564.2	416.6	299.2	203.5	154.2	124.2	62.9	42.1	31.6	25.3	21.1	18.1	15.9
135	585.9	432.6	310.7	211.4	160.2	128.9	65.3	43.7	32.9	26.3	21.9	18.8	16.5
140	607.6	448.6	322.2	219.2	166.1	133.7	67.7	45.3	34.1	27.3	22.8	19.5	17.1
145	629.3	464.6	333.7	227.0	172.0	138.5	70.1	47.0	35.3	28.3	23.6	20.2	17.7
150	651.0	480.7	345.2	234.9	178.0	143.3	72.5	48.6	36.5	29.2	24.4	20.9	18.3

Table 2-12. Ideal Body Weight (IBW) vs Actual Body Weight (ABW) for CD34+ Cell Dosing*

To Estimate IBW:

For height in inches

Male IBW = 50 kg + 2.3 kg [Height (inches) – 60]
Female IBW = 45.5 kg + 2.3 kg [Height (inches) – 60]

For height in centimeters

Male IBW = 50 kg + 2.3 kg $\frac{[\text{Height (cm)} - 60]}{2.54}$

Female IBW = 45.5 kg + 2.3 kg $\frac{[\text{Height (cm)} - 60]}{2.54}$

*Used with permission from Brecher ME, Hay SN. Collected questions and answers. 9th ed. Bethesda, MD: AABB, 2008:62-3.

Table 2-13. Sickle Cell Calculations and Hemoglobin S Percentages*

Calculation of the volume to be exchanged:

*Goal: Hb S <30%, Hb A >70%, Final Hct of ~30%

$V_{ex} = BV \times \ln(S_i/S_f)$

where Vex = volume exchanged, BV = Blood volume, ln = natural logarithm, Si = the initial sickle Hb percentage, and Sf = the final sickle Hb percentage.

Example 1: SCD patient BV = 5 L, Hct 32%, Hb S = 100%
$V_{ex} = 5000 \text{ mL} \times \ln(100\%/30\%) = 6020 \text{ mL}$
To maintain patient's Hct: $6020 \text{ mL} \times 0.32 = 1926 \text{ mL or } \sim 9.6 \text{ units}$

Example 2: SCD patient with recent transfusion so Si does not = 100%
Weight = 34 kg, Hct 23.7%, Hb S = 86%, transfused with 1 unit RBCs
$BV = \times 34 \text{ kg} \times 70 \text{ mL/kg} = 2380 \text{ mL}$

Thus, patient's initial volume of RBCs would be 2380 mL × 0.237 (Hct) = 564 mLs of RBCs of which 86% would be sickle cells: 564 ×0.86 = 485 mL of sickle cells

If you assume 1 unit = 200 mL Hb A red cells, then the Hb S % in this patient after the transfusion of 1 unit of RBCs =
Volume of sickle cells/total volume of red cells = 485/(564 + 200) = 63.5%

*Used with permission from Brecher ME. Collected questions and answers. 8th ed. Bethesda, MD: AABB, 2004:72. SCD = sickle cell disease.

Table 2-14. Number of RBC Units Needed for Exchange in a Sickle Cell Patient

For example, given a patient starting and ending at a hematocrit of 30%, the table calculating the number of units for the exchange would look like the following:

Blood Volume (mL)

Percent HbS	3000	3500	4000	4500	5000	5500	6000	6500	7000
10	10.4	12.1	13.8	15.5	17.3	19.0	20.7	22.5	24.2
20	7.2	8.4	9.7	10.9	12.1	13.3	14.5	15.7	16.9
30	5.4	6.3	7.2	8.1	9.0	9.9	10.8	11.7	12.6
40	4.1	4.8	5.5	6.2	6.9	7.6	8.2	8.9	9.6
50	3.1	3.6	4.2	4.7	5.2	5.7	6.2	6.8	7.3
60	2.3	2.7	3.1	3.4	3.8	4.2	4.6	5.0	5.4
70	1.6	1.9	2.1	2.4	2.7	2.9	3.2	3.5	3.7
80	1.0	1.2	1.3	1.5	1.7	1.8	2.0	2.2	2.3
90	0.5	0.6	0.6	0.7	0.8	0.9	0.9	1.0	1.1

Used with permission from Brecher ME, Shulman I. Collected questions and answers. 10th ed. Bethesda, MD: AABB, 2011.

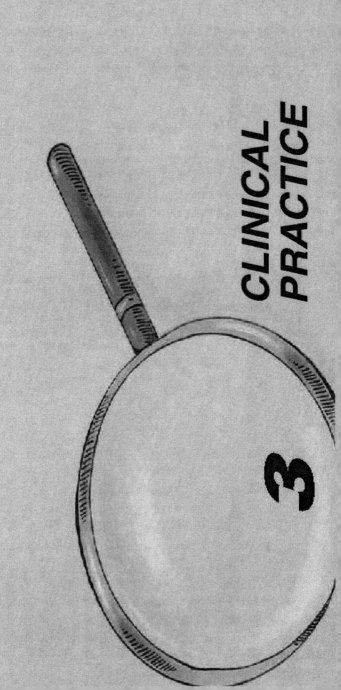

CLINICAL PRACTICE

3

Table 3-1. Effects of Plasma Exchange on Selected Medications*†

Examples of Drugs That Typically Do Not Need Dose Adjustment	Examples of Drugs That Are Removed and May Need Supplemental Dosages or Administration Timing Changes
Acetaminophen	Alemtuzumab (Campath)
Acyclovir	Amlodipine
Amiodarone	Ampicillin
Amlodipine	Basiliximab (Simulect)
Azathioprine	Ceftriaxone‡
Carbamazepine	Chloramphenicol
Cefepime	Cisplatin
Ceftazidime	Dalteparin
Cyclophosphamide	Diclofenac
Cyclosporine§	Diltiazem
Dapsone	Gentamycin
Digoxin/Digitoxin	Infliximab (Remicade)
Disopyramide	Interferon alpha
Mycophenolic acid‡	Intravenous immune globulin

Oxcarbazepine
Phenobarbital
Phenytoin
Prednisone/Prednisolone
Quinine
Tacrolimus[§][*]
Valproic acid
Vancomycin
Zidovudine

Palivizumag (Synagis)
Proxyphene
Propranolol
Rituximab
Theophylline
Thyroxin
Tobramycin
Teicoplanin
Trastuzumab
Verapamil
Vincristine

*Adapted with permission from Introduction to therapeutic apheresis: Principles, physiology, and patient management. In: Winters JL, King K, eds. Theraputic apheresis: A physician's handbook. 4th ed. Bethesda, MD: AABB, 2013 (in press).
See also: Ibrahim RB, Balogun RA. Medications in patients treated with therapeutic plasma exchange: Prescription dosage, timing, and drug overdose. Semin Dial 2012;25:176-89.
[†]Infusion of any drug just before or during an apheresis treatment should be avoided when possible.
[‡]Might be removed if dose given within 3 to 4 hours.
[§]Would be removed with red cell exchange.

Table 3-2. Key Medical Decisions in Therapeutic Apheresis*

Rationale and appropriateness of treatment

- Are there alternative diagnoses?
- What is the disease pathogenesis?
- Is there published experience with therapeutic apheresis for this indication?
- Which modality of therapeutic apheresis is appropriate?
- Is therapeutic apheresis effective?
- Is therapeutic apheresis the primary treatment?
- What is the likelihood that the disease will respond?
- What are the alternatives to therapeutic apheresis?
- Is therapeutic apheresis indicated now (can it wait)?
- What is the risk-to-benefit ratio of therapeutic apheresis?

Patient assessment and monitoring

- What is the patient's clinical status (renal/fluid balance, cardiovascular function, pulmonary function, coagulation)?
- Can the patient tolerate the procedure? Give informed consent?
- Where should the procedure be performed?

Treatment plan and endpoint

- What kind of vascular access is indicated?

- What is the proper "dose" per treatment?
- What is the proper number of treatments? What frequency?
- What comorbid conditions might alter the protocol?
- Can the patient tolerate the proposed extracorporeal volume and intraprocedure hematocrit?
- What type of replacement fluids should be prescribed?
- Which baseline laboratory tests are most relevant?
- Will any of the patient's current medications interfere with therapeutic apheresis?
- Will therapeutic apheresis remove or interfere with concurrent medications? Interfere with other treatments? Affect the accuracy of subsequent diagnostic tests?
- Is any pretreatment medication needed? Any medication during treatment?
- Will any special monitoring be needed during or after treatment?
- What parameters will be followed to assess the efficacy of treatment?
- What is the endpoint of the treatment plan?
- Who is responsible for care of the access line during and after the treatment course?

*Used with permission from Winters JL, King K, eds. Therapeutic apheresis: A physician's handbook. 4th ed. Bethesda, MD: AABB, 2013.

137

Table 3-3. Guidelines for Physicians Overseeing TA*

Position	Criteria
Medical director	• A licensed physician, qualified by training and/or by experience, who will be called the medical director in these Guidelines, should oversee each therapeutic apheresis (TA) service.
	• Apheresis therapy is best provided by the medical director, or a qualified designee, as a consultative service to an individual patient.
	• To act as the leader of the TA service and as a consultant to other physicians, the medical director should possess the following qualifications:
	– Detailed knowledge of relevant concepts in immunology and transfusion medicine, and of the basic principles of separation and transfusion of blood components and their physiologic renewal after removal or exchange
	– Operational familiarity with the specific instruments used by the TA service
	– Detailed knowledge of the diseases treated by TA and the clinical indications for TA in these diseases; familiarity with current relevant literature [eg, current edition of the American Society for Apheresis (ASFA) guidelines on the use of TA]
	– Expertise in the different applications of current modalities of apheresis therapy
	– Expertise in the management of adverse effects of TA

138

- Familiarity with the logistic, financial, and personnel issues involved in the management of a TA service

• Physicians who presently function as directors of TA services and have acquired such expertise by accumulated experience prior to January 1, 2005, are not subject to criteria listed below.

• Newly appointed medical directors will generally be considered qualified if they:

  - Have documented training in apheresis in relevant accredited postgraduate medical education (eg, transfusion medicine, hematology/oncology, nephrology, clinical pathology); AND/OR

  - Have documented participation in continuing education specifically related to TA offered by ASFA, the AABB, or equivalent organizations; AND

  - Are board certified or board eligible; AND

  - Have participated in a minimum of 50 TA procedures involving 15 different patients (note: participation should be documented)

• Physicians who are appointed as medical directors with no documentation of prior training and/or experience will not be considered qualified under these Guidelines.

(cont'd)

Table 3-3. Guidelines for Physicians Overseeing TA* (Continued)

Position	Criteria
	• Medical directors of TA services that serve more than one facility, including mobile TA Services, should be members of the staff at all medical facilities served by their teams in order to provide consultation. However, due to local regulations and credentialing requirements, such arrangements may not be always feasible or practical. If the director of the TA service is not credentialed in the facility, a designated physician on staff at the facility (see below for qualified designee) should be responsible for the immediate direct care patient management. In such situations, the medical director of the TA service should be available for consultation.
Qualified designee overseeing TA procedures	• Designated on-site physicians should receive formal documented training according to written policies/standard operating procedures in the TA service. This structured training should include the observation of a minimum of 10 TA procedures involving 5 different patients for which the designated physician does not have management authority (such as those performed at the director's home facility).
	• On-site designees overseeing TA procedures who do not have training and/or experience are not considered qualified under these Guidelines.

Additional support staff (eg, mobile apheresis services)

- After formulating the apheresis medicine treatment plan with the requesting physician by consultation, the director, or his/her designee, may delegate authority for immediate oversight and management of the patient to the requesting physician who does not have specialized training in apheresis. Documentation in the apheresis medicine record should reflect this clinical delegation. Such activities may include any or all of the following:
  - Ordering the procedure, including blood components and derivatives
  - Medications
  - Vascular access
  - Laboratory monitoring
  - Treatment of any adverse reactions

- The medical oversight of the procedure remains the responsibility of the requesting physician before, during, and after the procedure. Specific procedural oversight must be delegated to a physician (or his/her designee) with privileges at the facility where the procedure is going to take place and who is immediately available on-site—or if not, by telephone, as long as emergency medical services are immediately available on-site. If emergency medical services are not immediately available on-site, the physician overseeing the procedure must be available on-site. The director, or his/her qualified designee, must also be immediately available by telephone for consultation.

(cont'd)

Table 3-3. Guidelines for Physicians Overseeing TA* (Continued)

*Adapted with permission from the American Society for Apheresis (ASFA) (http://www.apheresis.org/~ASSETS/DOCUMENT/ GUIDELINES%20FOR%20PHYSICIANS%20OVERSEEING%20THERAPEUTIC%20APHERESIS%20.pdf). These Guidelines, developed by the Apheresis Applications Committee of ASFA, are intended to focus attention on two issues important in the quality of care: the recognition that a qualified physician is the best provider of therapeutic apheresis services and the importance of the maintenance of professional knowledge. These Guidelines were published on September 14, 2005 and reviewed and revised in January 2011. The Guidelines will be reviewed by the Board of Directors of ASFA bi-annually.

Disclaimer: It is the intent of ASFA), the authors and the editors, to provide current and accurate information to the reader. Furthermore, ASFA, the authors and the editors disclaim any responsibility for any adverse event as a consequence, directly or indirectly, from the application of any suggested treatment, protocol, and/or procedure. Nor will ASFA, the authors or the editors accept responsibility for any undetected errors or misunderstanding of any information contained in this document. The apheresis principles, policies, and procedures described in this document must be prescribed by a qualified physician and administered under the supervision of a qualified physician (as outlined in the ASFA publication Organizational Guidelines For Therapeutic Apheresis Facilities and the ASFA Clinical Applications and Standards Committee) and in accordance with applicable federal, state, and local regulatory agency requirements.

Table 3-4. Guidelines for Documentation of Therapeutic Apheresis Procedures in the Medical Record by Apheresis Physicians*

	Guidelines
Purpose	• These Guidelines are intended to assist medical establishments that maintain a therapeutic apheresis (TA) service with consultations that are provided with either direct or indirect medical intervention. • They are designed as a means to improve the quality of care and standardize the documentation of TA procedures. • An additional end result is to assist physicians with the documentation that is required for the various common procedural terminology (CPT) codes used to bill for physician services.
Physician's role	• As referenced by CPT codes (see below), TA procedures should be provided by physicians whose credentials satisfy the responsible institution's requirements for ordering and supervising such procedures (see Table 3-3). • These services are best provided as a consultative service to an individual patient. • The supervising physician is responsible for documenting his/her supervision of the apheresis procedure in the medical record according to the standards of the institution.

(cont'd)

Table 3-4. Guidelines for Documentation of Therapeutic Apheresis Procedures in the Medical Record by Apheresis Physicians* (Continued)

	Guidelines

Documentation	• The physician's procedure note should include documentation of at least the following points:
	  1. The physician reviewed and evaluated the pertinent clinical and laboratory data relevant to the treatment of the patient that day.
	  2. The physician has made the decision to perform the therapeutic procedure on the day in question.
	  3. The physician saw and evaluated the patient for the procedure.
	  4. The physician remained available to respond in person to emergencies or other situations requiring his/her presence throughout the duration of the procedure.
	• The four points establish that the procedure was carried out under the physician's supervision and under the physician's orders, and they serve as guidelines for a procedure note.
	• As described, the note does reference the fundamental clinical and laboratory data that the TA physician must take into account while managing a patient prior to and during a procedure.
	• These Guidelines do not specify how the four main points are to be documented; they only suggest the points that need to be properly referenced.

144

Documentation (continued)	• The four points do not address all of the elements required in an evaluation and management (E&M) note for coding and billing purposes, as defined in the fourth edition of the CPT by the American Medical Association. Apheresis physicians may also use E&M coding guidelines to document care delivered in the peri-treatment period.
CPT codes[†]	36511–Therapeutic apheresis for white cells
	36512–Therapeutic apheresis for red cells
	36513–Therapeutic apheresis for platelets
	36514–Therapeutic apheresis for plasmapheresis
	36515–Therapeutic apheresis with extracorporeal immunoadsorption and plasma reinfusion
	36516–Therapeutic apheresis with extracorporeal selective adsorption or selected filtration and plasma reinfusion

(cont'd)

Table 3-4. Guidelines for Documentation of Therapeutic Apheresis Procedures in the Medical Record by Apheresis Physicians* (Continued)

Guidelines
36522–Photopheresis, extracorporeal
38205–Blood-derived hematopoietic progenitor cell harvesting for transplantation per collection; allogeneic
38206–Blood-derived hematopoietic progenitor cell harvesting for transplantation per collection; autologous

*Adapted with permission from the American Society for Apheresis (ASFA; http://www.apheresis.org). These Guidelines were developed and published by the Apheresis Applications Committee of ASFA in September 2005. They were developed for acceptable documentation of the apheresis physician's services during a therapeutic procedure.

†For more information on billing practices, see "A Guide to Billing and Securing Appropriate Reimbursement, 2012 Edition" (Available at http://www.apheresis.org/~ASSETS/DOCUMENT/ASFA Therapeutic Apheresis Reimbursement Guide 2012 FINAL1.pdf).

Table 3-5. Example of an Apheresis Medicine Service Consultation Form*

Apheresis Medicine Service Consult to Initiate Therapeutic _____ **Procedures**

Patient Name: _____
Last, First, MI

Medical Record No.: _____

Date of Birth: ___/___/___

Location: _____

Attending Physician: _____
Last, First, MI

Contact Number/Pager: _____

Date of Consult: ___/___/___

Gender: ☐ Female ☐ Male

History obtained from: ☐ Patient ☐ Chart ☐ Family member ☐ Guardian ☐ Other:___

Chief Complaint:

History of Present Illness:

Past Medical History:

Current Medications (Be sure ACE inhibitors have been discontinued):

Medications Prior to Admission:

Allergies:

Social History:

Family History:

147

(cont'd)

Table 3-5. Example of an Apheresis Medicine Service Consultation Form* (Continued)

Review of Systems and Physical Exam:

Height: _____ Weight: _____ BP: _____ HR: _____ /min RR: _____ /min Temp: _____

Blood Volume: _____ mL Plasma Volume: _____ mL RBC volume for Exchange: _____ mL

General and Mental Status:

Neurologic:

Cardiac:

Pulmonary:

Renal:

Transfusion Service:

ABO: _____ Rh: _____ Antibody Screen: _____ Antibody ID: _____

DAT: _____ Polyspecific AHG: _____ Anti-IgG: _____ Anti-C3d: _____

Transfusion History (products and reactions):

Antigen Pheno(Geno)type for Sickle Cell patients:

Labs:

```
      Hb    Platelets              Schistocytes: _____
       \   /                              Na  |  Cl  |  BUN
WBC     \ /                               ----+------+-----  Glucose
  \     / \                                K  | HCO₃ |  Cr  /
   \   /   Hct                                              /
    \ /                                                    /
```

WBC   /\   Hb Platelets   Na | Cl | BUN Glucose
      / \ / \ /   K | HCO₃ | Cr

Schistocytes: _____

$$Na \mid Cl \mid BUN$$

PT: _____   INR: _____   PTT: _____   Fibrinogen: _____   ADAMTS13: _____

LDH: _____   Ionized Ca²⁺: _____   D-Dimer: _____   Haptoglobin: _____   ADAMTS13 Inhibitor: _____

Other Labs: _____

Vascular Access:

☐ Single or ☐ Dual access required

☐ Peripheral, antecubital fossa

☐ Central: ☐ right ☐ left and   Location: ☐ subclavian ☐ internal jugular ☐ femoral

☐ Other (describe): _____

(cont'd)

Table 3-5. Example of an Apheresis Medicine Service Consultation Form* (Continued)

Assessment and Plan: This is a ____ year-old ☐ male ☐ female with _____

✓ We plan to perform #__ of therapeutic ☐ Plasma Exchange (TPE) ☐ Red Cell Exchange (RCE) ☐ Leukocytapheresis (LCA) for removal of ____ cells ☐ Other: _____ procedures.

✓ Procedure parameters include:

☐ Each TPE will exchange ____ plasma volume(s) with ☐ 5% Albumin ☐ Plasma ☐ Albumin+Plasma and will maintain a ____ % fluid balance.

☐ The RCE and goal HCT ____% with fraction of cells remaining at ____ % fluid balance.

☐ The LCA goal of ____% reduction and/or to the ____ cell count of ____ with a ____ % fluid balance.

✓ The procedures are scheduled for the following dates:

And will take place in the following location:

✓ Please check the following labs in the morning of each procedure day:

☐ CBC ☐ PT/INR ☐ PTT ☐ Fibrinogen ☐ Ionized Calcium ☐ LDH ☐ _____

✓ Dr. _____ from the Apheresis Medicine Service discussed this plan with Dr. _____ from the _____ service on __/__/__ (date) at _____ (time).

✓ Dr. _____ has obtained the consent for _____ procedure(s). Risks, benefits, and alternative treatments were discussed with the patient, and questions were answered on __/__/__ (date). The signed consent form is in the patient's medical record. Consent for blood transfusion was obtained by Dr. _____ on __/__/__ (date) and is also in the medical record.

150

Resident/Fellow's Full Name: Print, Sign, and Date   Contact Number

Attending's Full Name: Print, Sign, and Date   Contact Number

(Courtesy of Gay Wehrli, MD, MSEd)

*Used with permission from Wehrli G. Transfusion therapy in therapeutic apheresis. In: Mintz PD. Transfusion therapy: Clinical principles and practice. 3rd ed. Bethesda, MD: AABB, 2011:394-5.
ACE = angiotensin-converting enzyme; AHG = antihuman globulin; DAT = direct antiglobulin test; Ig = immunoglobulin; INR = international normalized ratio; LDH = lactate dehydrogenase; PTT = partial thromboplastin time.

Table 3-6. Centrifugation-Based Therapeutic Apheresis Instruments*

Instrument	Procedures
COBE Spectra (Terumo BCT, Lakewood, CO)	TPE, RCE, RCD, WCC, WCD, PBSC, PC, PD, PS, MP
AS104[†] (Fresenius Kabi, Bad Homburg, Germany)	TPE, RCE, RCD, WCC, WCD, PBSC, PC, PD, PS, MP
COM.TEC (Fresenius Kabi, Bad Homburg, Germany)	TPE
UVAR XTS (Therakos, Exton, PA)	ECP
CELLEX (Therakos, Exton, PA)	ECP
Spectra Optia (Terumo BCT, Lakewood, CO)	TPE, PBSC
AMICUS (Fenwal, Lake Zurich, IL)	TPE

*Adapted with permission from Wehrli G. Transfusion therapy in therapeutic apheresis. In: Mintz PD. Transfusion therapy: Clinical principles and practice. 3rd ed. Bethesda, MD: AABB, 2011:363.

[†]Although the AS104 instrument is no longer available in the US, the disposable kits are still supported by Fresenius-Kabi.

ECP = extracorporeal photopheresis; MP = marrow processing; PBSC = peripheral blood stem cell processing; PC = platelet collection; PD = platelet depletion; PS = plasma separation for secondary column processing; RCD = red cell depletion; RCE = red cell exchange; TPE = therapeutic plasma exchange; WCC = white cell collection; WCD = white cell depletion.

Table 3-7. Apheresis Instrumentation Overview*

	Haemonetics		Fenwal		CaridianBCT	Fresenius	
	MCS/MCS Plus	PCS-2	AMICUS	Autopheresis C	COBE Spectra	AS 104	COM.TEC
Type of system	IFC	IFC	CFC	IFCF	CFC	CFC	CFC
Weight (lb)	56	56	345	105	389	319	286
Height × width × depth (inches)	26 × 21.5 × 21.5	26.5 × 21.5 × 21.5	60 × 20.5 × 32	59 × 17 × 10	59.5 × 27.6 × 27.9	75.6 × 24 × 27.8	55 × 24 × 26
ECV (approx): Total/RBCs (mL)	Variable 225 bowl 480 (38% Hct)- 359 (52% Hct)/ 180	Variable 225 bowl 480 (38% Hct)- 359 (52% Hct)/ 182-187	Double needle 210/60	200	Double needle (with LRS) 272/52	Double needle 175	Double needle 175
			Single needle 329 mL (max) 64 + Max cycle volume × Hct		Single needle 361/93	Single needle 285	Single needle 285
					Granulocyte 285/114	Granulocyte 120	Granulocyte 120

(cont'd)

153

Table 3-7. Apheresis Instrumentation Overview*(Continued)

	Haemonetics		Fenwal		CaridianBCT	Fresenius	
	MCS/MCS Plus	PCS-2	AMICUS	Autopheresis C	COBE Spectra	AS 104	COM.TEC
Monitors:							
Draw pressure	Yes	Yes	Yes	Yes	Yes	Yes	Yes
Return pressure	Yes	Yes	Yes	Yes	Yes	Yes	Yes
Air present	Yes	Yes	Yes	Yes	Yes	Yes	Yes
AC delivery	Yes	Yes	Yes	No	Yes	Yes	Yes
Centrifuge pressure	Yes	Yes	Yes	Yes	Yes	No	No
Leak detector	No	No	No	No	No	Yes	No
Blood warmer	No	No		No		No (centrifuge 36 C)	No (centrifuge 36 C)
Donor applications	Plasma, platelets	Plasma	Platelets (plasma by-product)(red cells by-product)	Plasma	Platelets, granulocytes (plasma by-product)	Platelets, granulocytes (plasma by-product)	Platelets, granulocytes (plasma by-product)

*Used with permission from Burgstaler EA. Current instrumentation for apheresis. In: McLeod BC, Weinstein R, Winters JL, Szczepiorkowski ZM, eds. Apheresis: Principles and practice. 3rd ed. Bethesda, MD: AABB, 2010:76.
AC = anticoagulant; CFC = continuous-flow centrifugation; ECV = extracorporeal volume; Hct = hematocrit; IFC = intermittent-flow centrifugation; IFCF = intermittent-flow centrifugation and filtration; LRS = leukocyte reduction system; Max = Maximum; RBCs = red blood cells; WB = whole blood.

Table 3-8. Column-Based Therapeutic Apheresis Modalities*

Instrument	Columns	Procedure Category	Blood Constituents Removed	Example Indications
Plasaut EZ (Asahi Kasei Kuraru Medical Co, Ltd, Tokyo, Japan)	Plasmaflo OP (Asahi)	WB-PSA	Plasma	TPE procedures or plasma separation for secondary column
	Cascadeflo (Asahi)	PL-DFPP (used with Plasmaflo OP)	High-molecular-weight plasma constituents	MM, cryoglobulinemia, arteriosclerosis obliterans, FH, etc
	Rheofilter (Asahi)	PL-DFPP (used with Plasmaflo OP)	Fibrinogen and high-molecular-weight plasma constituents	AMD and SSHL
	Immunosorba TR and PH (Asahi)	PL-IAA (used with Plasmaflo OP)	Antibodies and immune complexes	SLE, RA with vasculitis, CIDP, MG, GBS, etc
	Plasorba BR (Asahi)	PL-PAA (used with Plasmaflo OP)	Bile acid and bilirubin	Primary biliary cirrhosis and hyperbilirubinemia

(cont'd)

155

Table 3-8. Column-Based Therapeutic Apheresis Modalities* (Continued)

Instrument	Columns	Procedure Category	Blood Constituents Removed	Example Indications
LIFE 18 Apheresis Unit (Miltenyi Biotec, Gladbach, Germany)	Cellsorba (Asahi)	WB-LCA	Granulocytes, monocytes, and lymphocytes	UC and CD
	LIFE 18 – Disk Separator (Miltenyi)	WB-PSA	Plasma	TPE procedures or plasma separation for secondary column
	TheraSorb LDL and LDL 100 Adsorber (Miltenyi)	PL-PAA (used with LIFE 18 – Disk Separator)	LDL-C, IDL-C and LP(a)	Homozygous or heterozygous FH, etc
	TheraSorb Ig and Ig Flex Adsorber (Miltenyi)	PL-IAA (used with LIFE 18 – Disk Separator)	Immunoblogulins (IgG, IgM, IgE and IgA) and immune complexes	ITP, SLE, MG, GBS, MS, DCM, AHR, etc
	TheraSorb Rheo Adsorber (Miltenyi)	PL-PAA (used with LIFE 18 – Disk Separator)	Fibrinogen and CRP	AMD, SSHL, PARD, etc

156

		WB-PSA	Plasma	Plasma separation for secondary column
Art Universal (Fresenius, Bad Homburg, Germany)	PlasmaFlux P2 dry – integrated plasma filter			
COM.TEC† (Fresenius, Bad Homburg, Germany) for plasma separation with ADAsorb (Medicap Clinic GmbH, Ulrichstein, Germany) column monitoring system or	Immunosorba (Fresenius)	PL-IAA	Immunoglobulins (mainly IgG) and immune complexes	GBS, MG, CIDP, SLE, RPGN, DCM, AHR, etc
Art Universal used with PlasmaFlux P2 dry (Fresenius)	Globaffin (Fresenius)	PL-IAA	Immunoglobulins (mainly IgG) and immune complexes	GBS, MG, CIDP, SLE, RPGN, DCM, AHR, etc
Art Universal (Fresenius, Bad Homburg, Germany)	MONET (Fresenius)	PL-DFPP (used with PlasmaFlux P2 dry)	High-molecular-weight plasma constituents: Fibrinogen, β_2-M, IgM, vWF, LDL-C, VLDL, and LP(a)	No specified indications provided in written material; homozygous or heterozygous FH (Fresenius, personal communication)

(cont'd)

Table 3-8. Column-Based Therapeutic Apheresis Modalities* (Continued)

Instrument	Columns	Procedure Category	Blood Constituents Removed	Example Indications
Art or Art Universal (Fresenius, Bad Homburg, Germany)	DALI (Fresenius)	WB-LDLA	LDL-C and LP(a)	Homozygous or heterozygous FH
Adamonitor (JIMRO, Ltd, Takasaki, Japan)	Adacolumn (JIMRO)	WB-LCA	Granulocytes and monocytes/macrophages	UC, CD, RA, SLE, and Behcet disease
MA-01† or MA-03‡‡ (Kaneka Corporation, Osaka, Japan)	Sulflux KP-05† (Kaneka)	WB-PSA	Plasma	Plasma separation for secondary column
	Liposorber LA-15† (Kaneka)	PL-PAA (used with Sulflux KP-05)	Apolipoprotein-B containing lipoproteins [LDL-C, LP(a), TG, and HDL]	Homozygous or heterozygous FH (PARD and FSGS in Japan)

158

Centrifugation-based instrument for plasma separation	Selesorb (Kaneka)	PL-PAA (used with Sulflux KP-05)	Anti-DNA, anti-cardiolipin antibody, and immune complexes	SLE
	Liposorber LA-40S (Kaneka)	PL-PAA	Apolipoprotein-B containing lipoproteins [LDL-C, LP(a), TG, and HDL]	Homozygous or heterozygous FH (PARD and FSGS in Japan)
MA-03 (Kaneka Corporation, Osaka, Japan) or DX-21 (Nikkiso Co, Ltd, Tokyo, Japan)	Liposorber D (DL-50, DL-75 and DL-100) (Kaneka)	WB-LDLA	Apolipoprotein-B containing lipoproteins [LDL-C, LP(a), TG, and HDL]	Homozygous or heterozygous FH
Used in conjunction with a dialysis instrument	Lixelle S-15, S-25, S-35 (Kaneka)	WB-AA	β_2-M	Dialysis-related amyloidosis

(cont'd)

Table 3-8. Column-Based Therapeutic Apheresis Modalities* (Continued)

Instrument	Columns	Procedure Category	Blood Constituents Removed	Example Indications
HELP System[†] (B. Braun, Bethlehem, PA)	Four integrated columns: 1. Plasma separator 2. Precipitate filter 3. Heparin adsorber 4. Dialysis ultrafilter	WB-LDLA	Apolipoprotein-B containing lipoproteins [LDL, LP(a), TG, and HDL], fibrinogen, and CRP	Homozygous or heterozygous FH
Used with a dialysis instrument plus plasma pump or with a CRRT instrument	Plasmaflo AP-05H(L)[†] (Asahi)	WB-PSA	Plasma	TPE procedures
Prisma CRRT System[§] (Gambro, Lakewood, CO)	Prisma TPE 2000 set[§] (Gambro, Lakewood, CO)	WB-PSA	Plasma	TPE procedures

Prismaflex† CRRT System (Gambro, Lakewood, CO)	Prismaflex TPE 1000 and 2000 sets‡ (Gambro Lundia AB, Lund, Sweden)	WB-PSA	Plasma	TPE procedures

*Used with permission from Wehrli G. Transfusion therapy in therapeutic apheresis. In: Mintz PD. Transfusion therapy: Clinical principles and practice. 3rd ed. Bethesda, MD: AABB, 2011:365-6.

†Food and Drug Administration approved and available in the United States.

‡MA-03 tubing kits and Prismaflex TPE sets have not been FDA approved.

§Although the Prisma instrument is no longer available for purchase in the United States, the disposable tubing sets are still supported by Terumo BCT.

AA = amyloidosis apheresis; AHR = acute humoral rejection; AMD = age-related macular degeneration; β_2-M = β_2-microglobulin; CD = Crohn disease; CIDP = chronic inflammatory demyelinating polyneuropathy; CRP = C-reactive protein; CRRT = continuous renal replacement therapy; DCM = dilated cardiomyopathy; DFPP = double filtration plasmapheresis; FH = familial hypercholesterolemia; FSGS = focal segmental glomerulosclerosis; GBS = Guillain-Barré syndrome; HDL = high-density lipoprotein; HELP = heparin-induced extracorporeal LDL-cholesterol precipitation; IAA = immunoadsorption apheresis; IDL = intermediate-density lipoprotein; Ig = immunoglobulin; ITP = idiopathic thrombocytopenic purpura; LCA = leukocytapheresis; LDLA = low-density lipoprotein apheresis; LDL-C = low-density lipoprotein cholesterol; LP = lipoprotein; MG = myasthenia gravis; MM = multiple myeloma; MS = multiple sclerosis; PAA = plasma adsorption apheresis; PS = plasma separator; PARD = peripheral artery disease; PL = plasma; PSA = plasma separation apheresis; RA = rheumatoid arthritis; SLE = systemic lupus erythematosus; SSHL = sudden sensorineural hearing loss; TG = triglycerides; TPE = therapeutic plasma exchange; TTP = thrombotic thrombobocytopenic purpura; UC = ulcerative colitis; vWF = von Willebrand factor; VLDL = very low-density lipoprotein; WB = whole blood.

Table 3-9. Complications of Therapeutic Apheresis and Suggested Management*

Type of Complication	Signs and Symptoms	Suggested Management
Procedure Related		
Anxiety with hyperventilation	Tachycardia, hypertension or hypotension, tingling of fingers and/or toes, diaphoresis	Have patient breathe into a paper bag. Offer supportive, calm reassurance. For hypotensive patients, place in Trendelenburg and administer normal saline bolus. Consider anxiolytics for subsequent procedures.
Vasovagal reaction	Bradycardia, hypotension, diaphoresis, pallor and nausea	Place patient in Trendelenburg, give normal saline bolus. Place cool moist towels on forehead. Stimulate patient. Consider ammonia spirits.
Hypocalcemia	Paresthesias, initially circumoral but may progress to involve other parts of body; vibration in jaw; nausea, vomiting, and diarrhea; chest tightness; hypotension; prolonged QT interval on EKG; tetany	Pause procedure. Slow citrate infusion by decreasing whole blood flow rate or increasing WB:ACD ratio. Administer calcium, either oral or IV. Add calcium to colloid or crystalloid replacement fluid for continuous replacement procedures (do not add calcium to plasma).

	Signs and Symptoms	Action
Hypovolemia or antihypertensive therapy	Hypotension, diaphoresis, tachycardia (the latter may not occur in patients on beta blockers)	Place patient in Trendelenburg, and give normal saline bolus. For subsequent procedures, increase colloid replacement, decreasing crystalloid replacement when applicable; consider holding antihypertensive dose until after apheresis, when applicable.
ACE inhibitor use	Flushing, hypotension	Hold apheresis for 24 to 48 hours after last ACE inhibitor dose.
Reaction to ethylene oxide	Burning eyes, periorbital edema, other allergic symptoms	Stop procedure; if feasible, perform double prime for subsequent procedures.
Replacement Fluid Related		
Allergic	Itching, urticaria, facial edema, change in voice, difficulty swallowing, wheezing, shortness of breath, hypotension	Administer IV diphenhydramine, IV methylprednisolone, and/or subcutaneous epinephrine.
Transfusion reaction (including nonhemolytic febrile, allergic, acute hemolytic, TRALI, etc)	Signs and symptoms will vary based on type of transfusion reaction but include fever (nonhemolytic febrile), itching, hives and wheezing (allergic), respiratory compromise	Stop infusion of blood product and follow transfusion reaction protocol.

(cont'd)

163

Table 3-9. Complications of Therapeutic Apheresis and Suggested Management* (Continued)

Type of Complication	Signs and Symptoms	Suggested Management
Vascular Access Related		
Sepsis	Hypotension, positive blood cultures	Treat patient with appropriate antimicrobials, hold apheresis until new catheter is placed, and use peripheral access if feasible.
Thrombosis	Catheter cannot be flushed, high-pressure alarms indicate suboptimal flow	Radiograph to assess placement if appropriate; instill thrombolytic agent.

*Used with permission from Chhibber V, King KE. Management of the therapeutic apheresis patient. In: McLeod BC, Weinstein R, Winters JL. Szczepiorkowski ZM, eds. Apheresis: Principles and practice. 3rd ed. Bethesda, MD: AABB, 2010:239-40.

ACD = acid-citrate-dextrose; ACE = angiotensin-converting enzyme; EKG = electrocardiogram; IV = intravenous; TRALI = transfusion-related acute lung injury; WB = whole blood.

Table 3-10. Most Common Adverse Events in Therapeutic Apheresis*

	Frequency (%)
Overall adverse event	4.8
First-time procedure	6.9
Repeat procedure	4.3
Procedure-specific reaction rates	
Erythrocytapheresis	10.0
Plasma exchange (plasma replacement)	7.8
Leukocytapheresis	5.7
Plasma exchange (no plasma)	3.4
Autologous stem cell collection	1.7

(cont'd)

Table 3-10. Most Common Adverse Events in Therapeutic Apheresis* (Continued)

	Frequency (%)
Reaction by type	
Transfusion reactions	1.6
Citrate-related nausea and/or vomiting	1.2
Hypotension	1.0
Vasovagal nausea and/or vomiting	0.5
Pallor and/or diaphoresis	0.5
Tachycardia	0.4
Respiratory distress	0.3
Tetany or seizure	0.2
Chills or rigors	0.2

*Used with permission from McLeod BC, Sniecinski I, Ciavarella D, et al. Frequency of immediate adverse effects associated with therapeutic apheresis. Transfusion 1999;39:282-8.

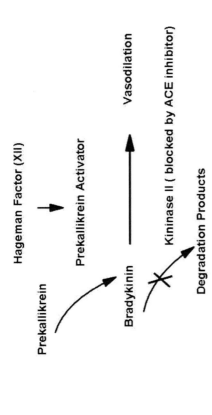

Figure 3-1. Angiotensin-converting enzyme (ACE) reaction mechanism. Prekallikrein activator (PKA) is found in small amounts in purified protein fraction (PPF) and albumin preparations. Used with permission from Brecher ME, Hay SN. Collected questions and answers. 9th ed. Bethesda, MD: AABB, 2008:28.

Table 3-11. Tests That Might Help Differentiate TTP from aHUS and Identify the Pathophysiology Associated with aHUS

ADAMTS13 activity, ADAMTS13 inhibitor assay

Serum levels of:
- C3
- C4
- Factor H
- Factor I

Screening for Factor H autoantibodies

Measurement of membrane cofactor protein (MCP, CD46) expression on peripheral blood mononuclear cells

Mutation screening of:
- CFH
- CFI
- CD46
- CFR
- C3
- THBD
- MCP

Screening for genomic disorders affecting CFH and CFHRs

Adapted from the following sources:

Kavanagh D, Goodship THJ. Atypical hemolytic uremic syndrome, genetic basis, and clinical manifestations. Hematology Am Soc Hematol Educ Program 2011;2011:15-20.

Taylor CM, Machin S, Wigmore S, et al, for a working party from the Renal Association, the British Committee for Standards in Haematology, and the British Transplantation Society. Clinical practice guidelines for the management of atypical haemolytic uraemic syndrome in the United Kingdom. Macclesfield, UK: British Transplantation Society, 2009. [Available at http://www.bts.org.uk/Documents/Guidelines/Active/0109 aHUS Clinical Practicctice Guidelines Version 4 (2).pdf (accessed January 28, 2013).]

Molecular Otolaryngology and Renal Research Laboratories. Atypical hemolytic-uremic syndrome panel. Iowa City, IA: University of Iowa, 2013. [Available at http://www.healthcare.uiowa.edu/labs/morl/aHUS Panel.htm (accessed January 28, 2013).]

Table 3-12. Examples of Drug Orders Useful in Therapeutic Apheresis*

Allergic prophylaxis or treatment

- Diphenhydramine (Benadryl): 25-50 mg by mouth 30 minutes before apheresis or IVP over 1-2 minutes (dilute in 10 mL of normal saline) for immediate action
- Hydroxyzine (Atarax): 10-30 mg by mouth 30 minutes before apheresis
- Ranitidine (Zantac): 150 mg by mouth 30 minutes before apheresis
- Nizatidine (Axid) 150-300 mg by mouth 30 minutes before apheresis
- Diphenhydramine (Benadryl) IV drip: 50-100 mg of diphenhydramine diluted in 100 mL of normal saline infused slowly over the interval of the procedure

Anaphylaxis

- Epinephrine 1:1000, 0.3-0.4 mL subcutaneously, may repeat in 10-15 minutes
- Methylprednisolone (Solu-Medrol) 1-2 mg/kg slow IVP

Citrate toxicity prophylaxis

- Calcium chloride ($CaCl_2$), 200 mg per liter of replacement in saline, HES, or albumin
- Calcium gluconate ($C_{12}H_{22}CaO_{14}$), 10 mL of 10% calcium gluconate per liter of return fluids: saline, HES, or albumin
- Calcium chloride ($CaCl_2$), 1 g diluted in 0.9% saline and infused at 200-300 mg/hour (50-75 mL/hour)

170

Citrate toxicity therapy

- Calcium carbonate ($CaCO_3$), eg, antacids as necessary for mild symptoms
- Calcium chloride ($CaCl_2$), 10%, 100-200 mg slow IVP over 2 minutes
- Calcium gluconate ($C_{12}H_{22}CaO_{14}$), small boluses of 10% by IV drip (up to 25 mL during a 3-5-L exchange)

Nausea

- Promethazine (Phenergan) by mouth, intramuscularly, or intravenously
  - 2-5 years of age: 5 mg
  - 5-10 years of age: 10 mg
  - Over 10 years of age: 25 mg
- Intravenously, promethazine hydrochloride should be given in concentration no greater than 25 mg/mL at a rate not to exceed 25 mg per minute

Sedation/anxiety

- Lorazepam (Alzapam, Ativan, Loraz, Lorazepam Intensol given intravenously, intramuscularly, or by mouth)
  - 18-60 years of age: 2-3 mg
  - Over 60 years of age: 0.5-1 mg

*Used with permission from Brecher ME, Hay S. Look It Up! (A quick reference in transfusion medicine). 2nd Ed. Bethesda, MD: AABB Press, 2012:98-9.
Unless otherwise indicated, all dosing is for adults.
HES = hydroxyethyl starch; IVP = intravenous push.

Table 3-13. Half-Lives of ACE-Inhibitor Drugs and Their Active Metabolites*

Generic Name	Brand Name	Parent Drug Half-Life (in hours)	Active Metabolite	Active Metabolite Half-Life (in hours)
Benazepril	Lotensin	0.6	Benazeprilat	10-11
Captopril	Capoten, Renitec	<3[†]		
Captopril and HCTZ	Capozide	<3[†]		
Enalapril	Vasotec		Enaliprilat	11
Enalapril and HCTZ	Vaseretic		Enaliprilat	11
Fosinopril sodium	Monopril, Fositen		Fosinoprilat	11.5-12
Imidapril	Tanatril	1.1-2.5	Imidaprilat	10-19
Lisinopril	Zestril, Prinivil, Listril, Lopril, Novatec	12[†]		
Lisinopril and HCTZ	Zestoretic, Prinzide	12[†]		
Moexipril	Univasc	1.3	Moexiprilat	12
Moexipril and HCTZ	Uniretic	1.3	Moexiprilat	12

Perindropil	Aceon, Acertil, Armix, Coverene, Coverex, Coversum, Coversyl, Covinace, Pericard, Prestarium, Prexanil, Prexum, Procaptan, Provinance	0.8-1		
Quinapril	Accupril	1-2	Quinaprilat	3
Quinapril and HCTZ	Accuretic	1-2	Quinaprilat	3
Ramipril	Altace	5.1	Ramiprilat	13-17[†]
Trandolapril	Mavik, Odrik, Gopten	6	Trandoaprilat	10
Zofenopril	Zofecard	0.9	Zofenoprilat	3.6-5.5

*Adapted with permission from Brecher ME, Hay SN. Collected questions and answers. 9th ed. Bethesda, MD: AABB, 2008:30.

[†]May be increased in renal failure.

Possible alternative medications include the following angiotensin II receptor antagonists: losartan (Cozaar), candesartan (Atacand), valsartan (Diovan), irbesartan (Avapro), telmisartan (Micardis), eprosartan (Teveten), olmesartan (Benicar), azilsartan (Edarbi).

ACE = angiotensin-converting enzyme; HCTZ = hydrochlorothiazide.

Table 3-14. Comparison of Replacement Fluids*

Replacement Solution	Advantages	Disadvantages
Crystalloids	Low cost Nonallergenic No viral risk	2-3 volumes required Hypo-oncotic Lacks coagulation factors and immunoglobulins
Albumin	Iso-oncotic Low risk of reactions	Higher cost Lacks coagulation factors and immunoglobulins
Plasma	Iso-oncotic Normal levels of coagulation factors, immunoglobulins, and other plasma proteins	Virus transmission risk Citrate load ABO compatibility required Risk of allergic reactions
Cryoprecipitate-reduced plasma	Iso-oncotic Reduced high-molecular-weight von Willebrand factor Normal levels of most other plasma proteins	Same as plasma

*Adapted with permission from Davenport RD. Therapeutic apheresis. In: Roback JD, Grossman BJ, Harris T, Hillyer CD, eds. Technical Manual. 17th ed. Bethesda, MD: AABB, 2011:718

174

Table 3-15. Alteration in Blood Constituents after One Plasma Volume Exchange

Constituent	Approximate Fraction Removed
Fibrinogen (rate-limiting factor)	2/3*
Immunoglobulins (IgM > IgG)	2/3*
Cholesterol	2/3*
Clotting factors	1/4 to 1/2
Paraproteins	1/3 to >1/2
Liver enzymes	>1/2
Bilirubin	~1/2

*May remain decreased after 48 hours.
IgM = immunoglobulin M; IgG = immunoglobulin G.
Reprinted with permission from Winters JL, King K, eds. Therapeutic apheresis: A physician's handbook. 4th ed. Bethesda, MD: AABB, 2013.

Table 3-16. Use of Therapeutic Plasma Exchange in Medication Overdose and Toxic Substances*

Medication	P_b (%)	V_d (L/kg)	Metabolism	Excretion
Digitoxin	30	6-7	Stomach	Urine
Cisplatin	90	0.3	Liver	Urine
Vincristine	75	7.2	Liver	Feces
Verapamil†	90	4.5-7	Liver	Urine
Thyroxine†	99‡	ND	Liver	Feces
Antithymocyte globulin	NA	0.12	Liver/Spleen	NA
Phenprocoumon (warfarin derivative)	99	0.14-0.17	Liver	Urine
Phenytoin†	90-95	0.6-0.7	Liver	Bile/Urine
Paraquat	0	1.2-1.6	Liver	Urine
Methylparathion	>90	10	Liver	Urine/Feces
Sodium chlorate	NA	ND	Kidney	Urine
Amanita toxin	Low	ND	NA	NA
Ethylene glycol	?	0.83	Liver	Urine

*Adapted with permission from Szczepiorkowski ZM. TPE in renal, rheumatic, and miscellaneous disorders. In: McLeod BC, Price TH, Weinstein R, eds. Apheresis: Principles and practice. 2nd ed. Bethesda, MD: AABB Press, 2003:365-409.
†Reports describing failure of plasma exchange were also published.
‡P_b also reported as 25% to 30% in Winters JL, Pineda AA, McLeod BC, Grima KM. Therapeutic apheresis in renal and metabolic diseases. J Clin Apher 2000;15:53-73.
NA = not applicable; ND = not determined; P_b = protein binding; V = volume of distribution.

Table 3-17. Criteria for Severe Malaria*

Manifestation	Features
Cerebral malaria	Unarousable; coma not attributable to any other cause, with a Glasgow coma scale score ≤9, and coma should persist for at least 30 minutes after a generalized convulsion
Severe anemia	Hematocrit <15% or hemoglobin <5 g/dL in the presence of parasite count >10,000/μL
Renal failure	Urine output <400 mL/24 hours in adults (<12 mL/kg/24 hours in children) and a serum creatinine >265 μmol/L (>3.0 mg/dL) despite adequate volume repletion
Pulmonary edema and acute respiratory distress syndrome	Acute lung injury score is calculated on the basis of radiographic densities, severity of distress syndrome hypoxemia, and positive end-expiratory pressure
Hypoglycemia	Whole blood glucose concentration <2.2 mmol/L (<40 mg/dL)
Circulatory collapse	Systolic blood pressure <70 mm Hg in patients >5 years old or <50 mm Hg in children aged 1-5 years, with cold clammy skin or a core-skin temperature difference >10 C
Abnormal bleeding	Spontaneous bleeding from gums, nose, and/or gastrointestinal tract, or laboratory evidence of disseminated intravascular coagulation

(cont'd)

177

Table 3-17. Criteria for Severe Malaria* (Continued)

Manifestation	Features
Repeated generalized convulsions	≥3 convulsions observed within 24 hours
Acidemia/acidosis	Arterial pH <7.25 or acidosis (plasma bicarbonate <15 mmol/L)
Macroscopic hemoglobinuria	Hemolysis not secondary to glucose-6-phosphate dehydrogenase deficiency
Impaired consciousness	Rousable mental condition, prostration, or weakness
Hyperparasitemia	>5% parasitized erythrocytes or >250,000 parasites/μL (in nonimmune individuals)
Hyperpyrexia	Core body temperature >40 C
Hyperbilirubinemia	Total bilirubin >43 μmol/L (>2.5 mg/dL)

*Used with permission from Shaz B. Red cell exchange and other therapeutic alterations of red cell mass. In: McLeod BC, Weinstein R, Winters JL, Szczepiorkowski ZM, eds. Apheresis: Principles and practice. 3rd ed. Bethesda, MD: AABB, 2010:401.

Table 3-18. Indications for Red Cell Exchange in Malaria*

- Parasitemia >30% in the absence of clinical complications
- Parasitemia >10% in the presence of severe disease, especially cerebral malaria, acute renal failure, adult respiratory distress syndrome, jaundice, and severe anemia
- Parasitemia >10% and failure to respond to optimal chemotherapy after 12-24 hours
- Parasitemia >10% and poor prognostic factors (eg, elderly patient)

*Used with permission from Shaz B. Red cell exchange and other therapeutic alterations of red cell mass. In: McLeod BC, Weinstein R, Winters JL. Szczepiorkowski ZM, eds. Apheresis: Principles and practice. 3rd ed. Bethesda, MD: AABB, 2010:402.

Table 3-19. Patient Criteria for the Use of LDL Apheresis in Hypercholesterolemia

United States Food and Drug Administration	German Federal Committee of Physicians and Health Insurance Funds	International Panel on Management of FH	HEART-UK
• FH homozygotes with an LDL cholesterol >500 mg/dL (>13 mmol/L) • FH heterozygotes with an LDL cholesterol >300 mg/dL (>7.8 mmol/L) who have failed a 6-month trial of drug therapy in combination with an American Heart Association Step II diet	• FH homozygotes • Patients with severe hypercholesterolemia in whom maximal dietary and drug therapy for >1 year has failed to lower cholesterol sufficiently	• FH homozygotes • FH heterozygotes with symptomatic coronary artery disease in whom LDL cholesterol is >4.2 mmol/L or decreases by <40% with maximal medical management	• FH homozygotes in whom LDL cholesterol is reduced by <50% and/or is >9 mmol/L with drug therapy • FH heterozygotes or "bad family history" patients in whom there is objective evidence of progression of coronary disease and LDL cholesterol remains >5.0 mmol/L or decreases by <40% despite drug therapy

- FH heterozygotes with an LDL cholesterol >200 mg/dL (>5.2 mmol/L) and documented coronary artery disease who have failed a 6-month trial of drug therapy in combination with an American Heart Association Step II diet

- Individuals with progressive coronary artery disease, severe hypercholesterolemia, and Lp(a) >60 mg/dL in whom LDL cholesterol remains elevated despite drug therapy.

*Used with permission from Winters JL. Selective extraction of plasma constituents. In: McLeod BC, Weinstein R, Winters JL, Szczepiorkowski ZM, eds. Apheresis: Principles and practice. 3rd ed. Bethesda, MD: AABB, 2010:430.
FH = familial hypercholesterolemia; LDL = low-density lipoprotein; UK = United Kingdom.

Table 3-20. Comparison of Currently Available LDL Apheresis Systems*

System/Commercial Instrument	Method of LDL Removal	Substances Removed†	Advantages	Disadvantages
Dextran Sulfate				
Liposorber LA-15 (Kaneka, Osaka, Japan)	Binding to dextran sulfate on the basis of electrical charge	LDL: 56% to 65% HDL: 9% to 30% Triglycerides: 34% to 40% Lp(a): 52% to 61%	• Column can be regenerated	• System requires plasma separation • High hematocrit may interfere with plasma separation
Heparin-Induced Extracorporeal LDL Precipitation (HELP)				
Plasmat Secura and Plasmat Futura (Braun-Melsungen, Melsungen, Germany)	Precipitation of LDL by heparin at an acidic pH	LDL: 67% HDL: 15% Triglycerides: 41% Lp(a): 62%	• System removes fibrinogen	• High hematocrit may interfere with plasma separation • System is complicated

182

Method	Mechanism	Reduction	Advantages	Disadvantages
Double Filtration Plasmapheresis	Separation based on size by filtering plasma with a second filter	LDL: 56% HDL: 25% Triglycerides: 49% Lp(a): 53%	• System removes fibrinogen	• High hematocrit may interfere with plasma separation • System causes loss of some albumin, HDL, and IgG
Immunoadsorption Plasmaselect (Plasmaselect, Teterow, Germany)	Immobilized sheep apolipoprotein B-100 antibodies	LDL: 64% HDL: 14% Triglycerides: 42% Lp(a): 64%	• Column can be regenerated	• System causes exposure to animal proteins
Lipoprotein Hemoper-Fusion DALI (Fresenius Kabi AG, Bad Homburg, Germany)	Binding to polyacrylate-coated polyacrylamide beads on the basis of electrical charge	LDL: 61% HDL: 30% Triglycerides: 42% Lp(a): 64%	• Plasma separation is not necessary	• Column cannot be regenerated or reused

183

(cont'd)

Table 3-20. Comparison of Currently Available LDL Apheresis Systems*(Continued)

System/Commercial Instrument	Method of LDL Removal	Substances Removed[†]	Advantages	Disadvantages
Liposorber D (Kaneka)	Binding to dextran sulfate, covalently bonded to cellulose, on the basis of electrical charge	LDL: 62% HDL: 2.5% Triglycerides: 38% to 68% Lp(a): 56% to 72%	• Plasma separation is not necessary • Procedure time is shorter than Liposorber LA-15 • Protocol for reuse of columns has been published	• Column cannot be regenerated

*Used with permission from Winters JL. Selective extraction of plasma constituents. In: McLeod BC, Weinstein R, Winters JL, Szczepiorkowski ZM, eds. Apheresis: Principles and practice. 3rd ed. Bethesda, MD: 2010:432-3.

[†]Percentage removed in a typical treatment.

DALI = direct adsorption of lipoproteins; HDL = high-density lipoprotein; IgG = immunoglobulin G; LDL = low-density lipoprotein; Lp(a) = lipoprotein (a).

184

Table 3-21. Disorders Treated with Staphylococcal Protein A Columns*

PAS Column (Prosorba[†])	PAA Column (Immunosorba[‡])
Immune thrombocytopenic purpura[§]	Factor VIII inhibitors[§]
Rheumatoid arthritis[§]	Factor IX inhibitors[§]
Platelet alloimmunization	Antiglomerular basement membrane disease (Goodpasture syndrome)
Paraneoplastic CNS syndromes	Wegner granulomatosis
Papraproteinemic polyneuropathies	Focal segmental glomerulosclerosis
Chemotherapy-induced thrombotic thrombocytopenic purpura (eg, mitomycin-C)	Systemic lupus erythematosus
Malignancies unresponsive to conventional therapy	Myasthenia gravis
	Acute inflammatory demyelinating polyneuropathy (Guillain-Barré syndrome)
	Humoral rejection of solid organ transplants
	Autoimmune hemolytic anemia
	Dilated cardiomyopathy

* Used with permission from Winters JL. Selective extraction of plasma constituents. In: McLeod BC, Weinstein R, Winters JL, Szczepiorkowski ZM, eds. Apheresis: Principles and practice. 3rd ed. Bethesda, MD: 2010:418.
†Fresenius Kabi, Redmond, WA; PAS = protein A silica.
‡Fresenius Kabi AG, Bad Homburg, Germany; PAA = protein A agarose.
§Uses approved by the US Food and Drug Administration.
CNS = central nervous system; PAA = protein AA; PAS = protein AS.

185

Table 3-22. Nonbiologic Liver Support Systems*

System	Removal System	Substances Removed	Plasma or Whole Blood Treated?	Comments
Hemofiltration	Solutes and water are removed by filtration across a semipermeable membrane.	"Large"-molecular-weight substances	Whole blood	Does not remove small water-soluble toxins.
Hemodiafiltration	Mechanisms include both filtration across a membrane and dialysis to remove substances by diffusion.	"Large"- and "small"-molecular-weight substances	Whole blood	
Hemoperfusion	Charcoal, ion exchange resins, or proteins are used to bind toxins.	Water-soluble toxins	Whole blood	Has severe reactions caused by interactions between cellular elements and binding substances. Was abandoned in favor of hemoabsorption.

186

Hemodiabsorption	Charcoal, ion exchange resins, or proteins are used to bind toxins.	Water-soluble toxins	Plasma separated by plasmapheresis	Eliminates reactions seen with hemoperfusion and increases surface area for toxin adsorption.
Molecular adsorbents recirculating system (MARS)	A dialysate containing highly concentrated albumin uses diffusion to remove water-soluble toxins as well as toxins bound to albumin. The dialysate is then cleansed of water-soluble toxins against a bicarbonate buffer and albumin-bound toxins by hemodiabsorption with charcoal and ion exchange resin. The albumin dialysate is reused.	Water-soluble and albumin-bound toxins	Whole blood	Trials of MARS in treating ALF are ongoing.

*Used with permission from Pryor HI 2nd, Vacanti JP. The promise of artificial liver replacement. Front Biosci 2008;13:2140-59.
ALF = acute liver failure.

187

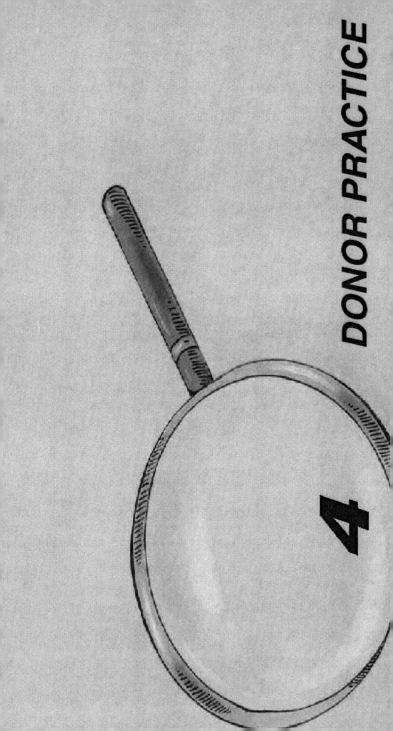

DONOR PRACTICE

4

Table 4-1. Requirements for Allogeneic Donor Qualification*†

Category	Criteria/Description/Examples	Deferral Period
1) Age	• Conform to applicable state law or • ≥16 years	
2) Whole Blood Volume Collected	• Maximum of 10.5 mL per kilogram of donor weight, including samples	
3) Donation Interval	• 8 weeks after whole blood donation (Standards 5.5.1-5.5.4 and 5.6.7.1 apply) • 16 weeks after 2-unit red cell collection • 4 weeks after infrequent plasmapheresis • ≥2 days after plasma-, platelet-, or leukapheresis	
4) Temperature	• ≤37.5 C (99.5 F) if measured orally, or equivalent if measured by another method	
5) Hemoglobin/ Hematocrit	• ≥12.5 g/dL/≥38%; blood obtained by earlobe puncture shall not be used for this determination • For double Red Blood Cell collections, follow instrument operator's manual	

6) Drug Therapy[‡]

Generic medication name [example of trade name(s)]

- Finasteride (eg, Proscar, Propecia), isotretinoin (eg, Accutane, Amnesteem, Claravis, Sotret)

  1 month after last dose

- Dutasteride (eg, Avodart)

  6 months after last dose

- Acitretin (eg, Soriatane)

  3 years after last dose

- Etretinate (eg, Tegison)

  Permanent

- Bovine insulin manufactured in the UK

  Indefinite

- Medications that irreversibly inhibit platelet function preclude use of the donor as sole source of platelets

  - Aspirin and piroxicam (eg, Feldene)

    2 full days (>48 hours) after last dose

  - Clopidogrel (eg, Plavix) and Ticlopidine (eg, Ticlid)

    14 days after last dose

- Warfarin (eg, Coumadin)

  For plasma products for transfusion: 1 week (7 days) after last dose

(cont'd)

191

Table 4-1. Requirements for Allogeneic Donor Qualification*† (Continued)

Category	Criteria/Description/Examples	Deferral Period
	• Heparin and derivatives • Direct thrombin inhibitors (eg, Dabigatran) • Direct Xa inhibitors (eg, Rivaroxaban)	For plasma products for transfusion: 1 week (7 days) after last dose or as defined by the facility's medical director
	• Receipt of Hepatitis B Immune Globulin	12 Months
	• Other medications, such as antibiotics	As defined by the facility's medical director
7) Medical History and General Health	• The prospective donor shall appear to be in good health and shall be free of major organ disease (eg, heart, liver, lungs), cancer, or abnormal bleeding tendency, unless determined suitable by the medical director • The venipuncture site shall be evaluated for lesions on the skin. The venipuncture site shall be free from infectious skin disease and any disease that might create a risk of contaminating the blood	

	Deferral Period
• Family history of Creutzfeldt-Jakob disease (CJD)§	Indefinite deferral for risk of CJD
8) Pregnancy	
• Defer if pregnant within the last 6 weeks	
9) Receipt of Blood, Blood Component, or Human Tissue	
• Receipt of dura mater or pituitary growth hormone of human origin	Indefinite
• Receipt of blood, components, human tissue, or plasma-derived clotting factor concentrates	12 months
10) Immunizations and Vaccinations	
• Receipt of toxoids, or synthetic or killed viral, bacterial, or rickettsial vaccines if donor is symptom-free and afebrile [Anthrax, Cholera, Diphtheria, Hepatitis A, Hepatitis B, Influenza, Lyme disease, Paratyphoid, Pertussis, Plague, Pneumococcal polysaccharide, Polio (Salk/injection), Rabies, Rocky Mountain spotted fever, Tetanus, Typhoid (by injection)]	None
• Receipt of recombinant vaccine [eg, HPV Vaccine]	
• Receipt of intranasal live attenuated flu vaccine	
• Receipt of live attenuated viral and bacterial vaccines [Measles (rubeola), Mumps, Polio (Sabin/oral), Typhoid (oral), Yellow fever]	2 weeks

(cont'd)

193

Table 4-1. Requirements for Allogeneic Donor Qualification*† (Continued)

Category	Criteria/Description/Examples	Deferral Period
	• Receipt of live attenuated viral and bacterial vaccines [German measles (rubella), Chicken pox (varicella zoster)]	4 weeks
	• Smallpox‖	Refer to FDA Guidance
	• Receipt of other vaccines, including unlicensed vaccines	12 months unless otherwise indicated by medical director
11) Infectious Diseases	• History of viral hepatitis after 11th birthday	Indefinite
	• Confirmed positive test for HBsAg¶	Permanent
	• Repeatedly reactive test for anti-HBc on more than one occasion	Indefinite#
	• Repeatedly reactive test for anti-HTLV on more than one occasion	Indefinite**
	• Present or past clinical or laboratory evidence of infection with HIV, HCV, HTLV, or *T. cruzi* or as excluded by current FDA regulations and recommendations for the prevention of HIV transmission by blood and components	Indefinite

194

- A history of babesiosis — Indefinite

- Evidence or obvious stigmata of parenteral drug use — Indefinite

- Use of a needle to administer nonprescription drugs — Indefinite

- Mucous membrane exposure to blood — 12 Months

- Nonsterile skin penetration with instruments or equipment contaminated with blood or body fluids other than the donor's own. Includes tattoos or permanent make-up unless applied by a state regulated entity with sterile needles and ink that has not been reused. — 12 Months

- Sexual contact or lived with an individual who: — 12 Months
  a. Has acute or chronic hepatitis B (positive HBsAg test, HBV NAT)
  b. Has symptomatic hepatitis C
  c. Is symptomatic for any other viral hepatitis

- Sexual contact with an individual with HIV infection or at high risk of HIV infection[††,‡‡] — 12 Months or as recommended by FDA

- Incarceration in a correctional institution (including juvenile detention, lockup, jail, or prison) for more than 72 consecutive hours — 12 Months

(cont'd)

Table 4-1. Requirements for Allogeneic Donor Qualification*† (Continued)

Category	Criteria/Description/Examples	Deferral Period

	• Syphilis or gonorrhea§§
	  a. Following the diagnosis of syphilis or gonorrhea. Must have completed treatment
	  b. Donor who has a reactive screening test for syphilis where no confirmatory testing was performed
	  c. A confirmed positive test for syphilis (FDA reentry protocol applies)
		12 months (in accordance with FDA Guidance)

	• West Nile virus	In accordance with FDA Guidance‖‖
	• Malaria¶¶ These deferral periods apply irrespective of the receipt of antimalarial prophylaxis: a. Prospective donors who have had a diagnosis of malaria	a. 3 years after becoming asymptomatic

	b. Individuals who have lived for at least 5 consecutive years in areas considered malaria-endemic by the Malarial Branch, Centers for Disease Control and Prevention, US Department of Health and Human Services	3 years after departure from malaria-endemic area(s)
	c. Individuals who have traveled to an area where malaria is endemic[##]	Defer for 12 months after departing that area
12) Travel	The prospective donor's travel history shall be evaluated for potential risks[§,‡‡,¶¶,##]	
	Donors recommended for deferral for risk of vCJD, as defined in most recent FDA Guidance[§]	Indefinite

---

*Adapted with permission from Carson TH, ed. Standards for blood banks and transfusion services. 28th ed. Bethesda, MD: AABB, 2012:55-60.

[†]For blood pressure, see 21 CFR 640.3(b)(2).

[‡]Medication Deferral List current version at http://www.aabb.org/resources/donation/questionnaires/Pages/dhqaabb.aspx.

[§]FDA Guidance for Industry, May 27, 2010, "Revised Preventive Measures to Reduce the Possible Risk of Transmission of Creutzfeldt-Jakob Disease (CJD) and Variant Creutzfeldt-Jakob Disease (vCJD) by Blood and Blood Products."

[‖]FDA Guidance for Industry, December 30, 2002, "Recommendations for Deferral of Donors and Quarantine and Retrieval of Blood and Blood Products in Recent Recipients of Smallpox Vaccine (Vaccinia Virus) and Certain Contacts of Smallpox Vaccine Recipients."

(cont'd)

197

Table 4-1. Requirements for Allogeneic Donor Qualification*† (Continued)

¶FDA Guidance for Industry, November 2011, "Requalification Method for Reentry of Donors Who Test Hepatitis B Surface Antigen (HBsAg) Positive Following a Recent Vaccination against Hepatitis B Virus Infection."

#FDA Guidance for Industry, April 30, 2010, "Requalification Method for Reentry of Blood Donors Deferred Because of Reactive Test Results for Antibody to Hepatitis B Core Antigen (Anti-HBc)."

**FDA Guidance for Industry, August 15, 1997, "Donor Screening for Antibodies to HTLV-II."

††FDA Memorandum, April 23, 1992, "Revised Recommendation for the Prevention of Human Immunodeficiency Virus (HIV) Transmission by Blood and Blood Products."

‡‡FDA Guidance for Industry, August 2009, "Recommendations for Management of Donors at Increased Risk for Human Immunodeficiency Virus Type I (HIV) Group O Infection."

§§FDA Memorandum, December 12, 1991, "Clarification of FDA Recommendations for Donor Deferral and Product Distribution Based on the Results of Syphilis Testing."

‖‖FDA Guidance for Industry, November 6, 2009, "Use of Nucleic Acid Tests to Reduce the Risk of Transmission of West Nile Virus from Donors of Whole Blood and Blood Components Intended for Transfusion."

¶¶FDA Memorandum, July 26, 1994, "Recommendations for Deferral of Donors for Malaria Risk."

#www.cdc.gov/travel.

FDA = Food and Drug Administration; HBsAg = hepatitis B surface antigen; HBV = hepatitis B virus; HCV = hepatitis C virus; HIV = human immunodeficiency virus; HPV = human papilloma virus; HTLV = human T-cell lymphotropic virus; NAT = nucleic acid testing; vCJD = variant Creutzfeld-Jakob disease.

Table 4-2. Malaria Risk—Federal Resources

Title	Agency	Internet	Comment
Travelers' health: Yellow book (2008)	Centers for Disease Control and Prevention	http://www.cdc.gov/travel/content YellowBook.aspx	Published every 2 years
Yellow fever vaccine requirements and information on malaria risk and prophylaxis, by country (2008)	Centers for Disease Control and Prevention	http://www.cdc.gov/travel/YellowBookCh5-Malaria YellowFeverTable.aspx	Chapter 5 in Yellow Book
Malaria risk world map	Centers for Disease Control and Prevention	http://www.cdc.gov/malaria/map	Beta version

Table 4-3. Automated Component Collection Instrument Overview

	CaridianBCT Trima Accel	Haemonetics		Fenwal	
		MCS+ LN 8150	Cymbal	ALYX	AMICUS
Type of system	IFD, CFC	IFC	IFC	IFD, CFC	IFD, CFC
Weight (lb)	185	56	29	51	345
Height × width × depth (inches)	41.9 × 20.8 × 32	26.5 × 21.5 × 21.5	14 × 14 × 20	26 × 18 × 19	75.6 × 24 × 27.8
ECV (approx):Without product Total	182-196	542 (38% Hct)-391 (54% Hct)	200 ml	110 + collect bags/ (110 × Hct) + (IP/ 1.05 g/mL) + RBCs/1.08 g/mL	329 ml (max)
Monitors:					
Draw pressure	Yes	Yes	Yes	Yes	Yes
Return pressure	Yes	Yes	Yes	Yes	Yes

Air present	Yes	Yes	Yes	Yes	Yes
AC delivery	Yes	Yes	Yes	Yes	Yes
Centrifuge pressure	Yes	Yes	Yes	Yes	Yes
Leak detector	Yes	Yes	Yes	Yes	Yes
Blood warmer	No	No	No	No	No
Donor applications	Plts (1 or 2 units) Concurrent plasma RBCs (1 or 2 units)	Concurrent plasma RBCs (1 or 2 units)	RBCs (2 units)	RBCs (1 or 2 units) Concurrent plasma	Plts (1 or 2 units) Concurrent plasma Concurrent RBCs (1 unit)

*Used with permission from Burgstaler EA. Current instrumentation for apheresis. In: McLeod BC, Weinstein R, Winters JL, Szczepiorkowski ZM, eds. Apheresis: Principles and practice. 3rd ed. Bethesda, MD: AABB Press, 2010:95.
AC = anticoagulant; CFC = continuous flow to centrifuge; ECV = extracorporeal volume; Hct = hematocrit; IFC = intermittent-flow centrifugation; IFD = intermittent flow to donor; IP = in-process bag; max = maximum; Plts = platelets; RBCs = red blood cells; WB = whole blood bag.

Table 4-4. Components That Can Be Collected from Various Instruments*

Instrument	GRAN	PLT	cRBC	2-RBC	PLASMA	cPLASMA
Fenwal ALYX			X	X		X
Fenwal Amicus		X	X			X
Fenwal Autopheresis C					X	
Fresenius AS104	X					
Caridian (COBE) Spectra	X	X				X
Caridian Trima V-4		X	X	X		X
Caridian Trima Accel		X	X	X		X
Haemonetics Cymbal				X		
Haemonetics MCS+ LN9000	X	X				X
Haemonetics MCS+ LN8150			X	X		X
Haemonetics PCS-2					X	

*Used with permission from Smith JW. Blood component collection by apheresis. In: Roback JD, Grossman BJ, Harris T, Hillyer CD, eds. Technical manual. 17th ed. Bethesda, MD: AABB, 2011:228.
Concurrent = more than one product can be collected; cPLASMA = concurrent plasma; cRBC = concurrent 1-unit RBC; GRAN = granulocytes; PLASMA = 1-unit plasma; PLT = plateletpheresis (single, double, triple); V-4 = software version 4; 2-RBC = double unit of RBCs.

202

Table 4-5. Timing and Red Cell Regeneration During Preoperative Autologous Donation*

Time from Donation to Surgery (days)	No. of Patients	Mean Red Blood Cell Units Regenerated	5% Confidence Interval of Mean
6-13	39	0.52	0.25-0.79
14-20	127	0.54	0.40-0.68
21-27	128	0.75	0.61-0.90
28-34	48	1.16	0.96-1.36
35-41	30	1.93	1.64-2.20

*Used with permission from Toy P, Ahn D, Bacchetti P. When should the first of two autologous donations be made? (abstract) Transfusion 1994;34(Suppl):14S.

Table 4-6. Simplified Allogeneic Red Cell Plus Plasma Donation Volumes*

Donor Weight (in lb)	Hematocrit (%)	Settings	
		Red Cells (mL)	Plasma (mL)
Males			
≥110 ≤ 129	≥38	185	450
	≥42	190	450
≥130 ≤ 149	≥38	195	500
	≥42	200	500
≥150 ≤ 174	≥38	210	550
	≥42	210	550
≥175	≥38	210	550
	≥42	210	550

Females		
≥110 ≤ 129	≥38	180	450
	≥42	185	450
≥130 ≤ 149	≥38	190	450
	≥42	195	450
≥150 ≤ 174	≥38	190	500
	≥42	195	550
≥175	≥38	200	550
	≥42	210	550

*Used with permission from Smith JW. Automated donations: Plasma, red cells, and multicomponent donor procedures. In: McLeod BC, Weinstein R, Winters JL, Szczepiorkowski ZM, eds. Apheresis: Principles and practice. 3rd ed. Bethesda, MD: AABB Press, 2010:135.

Table 4-7. Composition of Selected Platelet Additive Solutions (All values are expressed as mmol/L)*

	T-Sol[†]	InterSol[†]	Composol[‡]	SSP+[§]	PAS-G[**]	PAS-F[††]
NaCl	115.5	77.3	90	69.3	110	91
KCl	–	–	5	5	5	5
MgCl	–	–	1.5	1.5	3	1.5
Citric acid	–	–	–	–	7.5	–
Na citrate	10	10.8	11	10.8	–	–
Na acetate	30	32.5	27	32.5	15	27.2
Na bicarbonate	–	–	–	–	26.4	–
Na gluconate	–	–	23	–	–	–
Na phosphate	–	28.2	–	28.2	4	22.9
Glucose	–	–	–	–	30	0.5
K phosphate	–	–	–	–	–	0.1

*Modified with permission from Vassallo RR Jr, Murphy S. Apheresis platelet collection, storage, quality assessment, and clinical use. In: McLeod BC, Weinstein R, Winters JL, Szczepiorkowski ZM, eds. Apheresis: Principles and practice. 3rd ed. Bethesda, MD: AABB Press, 2010:155.
[†]Fenwal, Inc, Lake Zurich, IL.
[‡]Fresenius AG, Bad Homburg, Germany.
[§]Macopharma, Tourcoing, France.
[**]Pall Corp, East Hills, NY.
[††]Isoplate, B. Braun Medical, Irvine, CA.

206

Table 4-8. Simplified Allogeneic 2-Unit Red Blood Cell Donation Volumes for Donors of Different Weights*

Donor Weight (in lb)	Donor Height	Donor Hematocrit (%)	Absolute Red Cell Volume (mL)
Male			
130-149	≥5'1"	≥40	180 × 2
		≥42	190 × 2
150-174	≥5'1"	≥40	200 × 2
		≥42	210 × 2
175	≥5'1"	≥40	210 × 2
		≥42	210 × 2
Female			
150-174	≥5'5"	≥40	180 × 2
		≥42	190 × 2
175	≥5'5"	≥40	200 × 2
		≥42	210 × 2

*Used with permission from Smith JW. Automated donations: Plasma, red cells, and multicomponent donor procedures. In: McLeod BC, Weinstein R, Winters JL, Szczepiorkowski ZM, eds. Apheresis: Principles and practice. 3rd ed. Bethesda, MD: AABB Press, 2010:134.

207

Table 4-9. Requirements for Labeling Blood and Blood Components*

Item No.	Labeling Item	Collection or Preparation	Final Component	Pooled
1	Name of blood component or intended component[†]	NR	R	R
2	Donation identification number[†]	R	R	R
3	Identity of anticoagulant[‡] or other preservative solution	R	R	R
4	Identity of sedimenting agent, if applicable	NR	R	NA
5	Approximate volume[§]	NR	R	R, total
6	Facility collecting component[†]	NR	R	NR
7	Facility modifying component[||]	NA	R, if leaves the facility	R[†]
8	Storage temperature	NA	R	R
9	Expiration date and, when appropriate, time	NA	R	R
10	ABO group and Rh type[†,¶]	NA	R	See line 18
11	Specificity of unexpected red cell antibodies[#]	NA	R[‡]	R

208

No.				
12	Instructions to the transfusionist:	NR	R	R
	1. See *Circular of Information for the Use of Human Blood and Blood Components*			
	2. "Properly identify intended recipient"			
	3. "This product may transmit infectious agents"			
	4. "Rx Only"			
13	Phrase: "Volunteer Donor," if applicable	NR	R	R
14	Phrase: "Paid Donor," if applicable	R	R	R
15	CMV seronegative, if applicable	NR	R	R
16	Indication that the unit is low volume, and the actual volume, if applicable	NR	R	NA
17	Number of units in pool#	NA	NA	R
18	ABO and Rh of units in pool§,**	NA	NA	R
	Additional Autologous Labeling Requirements			
19	Phrase: "For autologous use only"	R	R	R
20	Recipient name, identification number, and, if available, name of facility where patient is to be transfused#	R	R	R

(cont'd)

Table 4-9. Requirements for Labeling Blood and Blood Components* (Continued)

Item No.	Labeling Item	Collection or Preparation	Final Component	Pooled
21	Biohazard label, if applicable[††]	NR	R	R
22	Phrase: "Donor untested," if applicable[‡‡]	NR	R	NA
23	Phrase: "Donor tested within the last 30 days," if applicable[§§]	NR	R	NA
	Additional Dedicated Donor Labeling Requirements			
24	Intended recipient information label	R	R	NA
25	Donor tested within the last 30 days, if applicable[§§]	NR	R	NA
26	Biohazard label, if applicable[††]	NR	R	R
	Labeling Requirements for Recovered Plasma[‖‖]			
27	"Caution: For Manufacturing Use Only"	NA	R	R
28	Biohazard label, if applicable	NR	R	R
29	"Not for Use in Products Subject to License Under Section 351 of the Public Health Service Act" (Applicable to plasma not meeting requirements for manufacture into licensable products)	NA	R	R

30	In lieu of expiration date, the date of collection of the oldest material in the container	R	R	R

*Adapted with permission from Carson TH, ed. Standards for blood banks and transfusion services. 28th ed. Bethesda, MD: AABB, 2012.

†Must be machine-readable (see Standard 5.1.6.3.1).

‡Not required for cryoprecipitate, frozen, deglycerolized, rejuvenated, or washed Red Blood Cells.

§For platelets, low-volume Red Blood Cells, Fresh Frozen Plasma, pooled components, and components prepared by apheresis, the approximate volume in the container.

‖Includes irradiation, if applicable.

¶Rh type not required for cryoprecipitate or pooled cryoprecipitate.

#The facility has the option of putting information on a tie tag or label. Specificity of antibodies is not required for autologous units.

**For pooled cryoprecipitate, plasma, or platelets of mixed types, a pooled type label is acceptable. The specific ABO group and Rh types of units in the pool may be put on a tie tag. Standard 5.7.4.3 applies.

(cont'd)

Table 4-9. Requirements for Labeling Blood and Blood Components* (Continued)

††Biohazard labels for autologous units or allogeneic units from a dedicated donor shall be used for the following test results:

Test	Test Result
HBsAg	Repeatedly reactive
Anti-HBc	Repeatedly reactive
Anti-HCV	Repeatedly reactive
HCV NAT	Positive or reactive
Anti-HIV-1/2	Repeatedly reactive
HIV-1 NAT	Positive or reactive
Anti-HTLV-I/II	Repeatedly reactive
WNV NAT	Positive or reactive
Syphilis	Reactive screening test with a positive confirmatory test or no confirmatory test

When performed:	
HBV NAT	Positive or reactive
T. cruzi Antibody Screening	Repeatedly reactive

‡‡Donor not tested for evidence of infectious diseases.
§§When the first unit has been tested but any unit collected within 30 days after the first collection has not been tested.
‖‖Labeling of Recovered Plasma shall conform to 21 CFR 606.121(e)(4) and 21 CFR 610.40(h)(2)(ii).

CMV = cytomegalovirus; HBc = hepatitis B core (antigen); HBsAg = hepatitis B surface antigen; HBV = hepatitis B virus; HCV = hepatitis C virus; HIV = human immunodeficiency virus; HTLV = human T-cell lymphotropic virus; NA = not applicable; NAT = nucleic acid amplification test (or technology); NR = not required; R = required; WNV = West Nile virus.

Table 4-10. Donor/Recipient HLA Match Grades (HLA-A and -B Antigens)*

Grade	Interpretation
A	All four donor antigens identical to those in recipient.
B1U	All donor antigens identical to those in recipient; only three antigens detected in donor (probable homozygous antigen).
B2U	All donor antigens identical to those in recipient; only two antigens detected in donor (probable homozygous haplotype).
B1X	Three donor antigens identical to those in recipient; the fourth is cross-reactive with a recipient antigen.
B2UX	Two donor antigens identical to those in recipient; a third is cross-reactive; only three antigens detected in donor (probable homozygous antigen).
B2X	Two donor antigens identical to those in recipient; two are cross-reactive.
C	One donor antigen is mismatched (not cross-reactive) with antigens in recipient.

*Adapted with permission from McFarland JG. Matched apheresis platelets. In: McLeod BC, Weinstein R, Winters JL, Szczepiorkowski ZM, eds. Apheresis: Principles and practice. 3rd ed. Bethesda, MD: AABB Press, 2010:188.

213

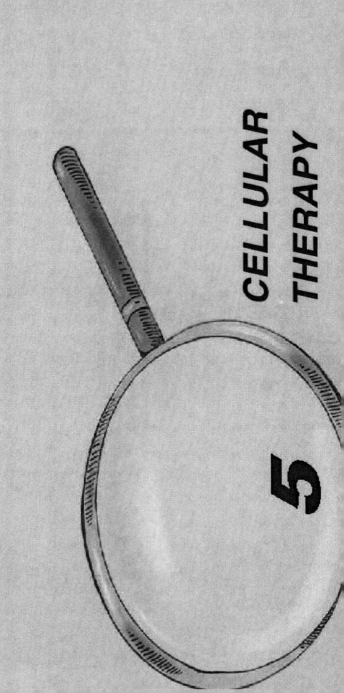

5

CELLULAR THERAPY

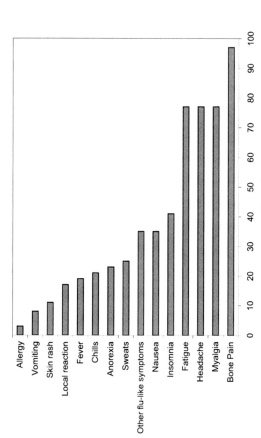

Figure 5-1. Signs and symptoms associated with granulocyte–colony-stimulating factor administration in healthy cellular therapy product donors. Percentage of 395 normal donors who experienced one or more signs or symptoms during mobilization of HPC-A using filgrastim, 5 to 10 μg/kg for 4 to 7 days, followed by apheresis. Data from National Marrow Donor Program. Used with permission from Lane T, McMannis JD. Hematopoietic progenitor cells collected by apheresis. In: Roback JD, Combs MR, Grossman BJ, Hillyer CD, eds. Core principles in cellular therapy. Bethesda, MD: AABB, 2008:25-46.

216

Table 5-1. General Requirements for fCellular Therapy Product Donors*†

I. Donor Advocacy Services

All living allogeneic donors shall be provided with the opportunity to access donor advocacy services.

II. Donor Education

A. The prospective donor [or legally authorized representative(s), if applicable] shall be provided with educational materials that describe the donation process and its potential risks and complications. The prospective donor [or legally authorized representative(s), if applicable] shall acknowledge in writing that he or she has read the educational material, has been given the opportunity to ask questions, and has had those questions answered satisfactorily.

B. Educational materials shall include the following elements:
   1) General explanation of the indications for and results of cellular therapy.
   2) General description of the donation process, donation alternatives, and the risks of donation.
   3) For marrow donors:
       a) Risks of anesthesia.
       b) Risks and discomforts of marrow donation, including infection, mechanical injury, and transfusion.
   4) For apheresis donors:
       a) Detailed information about the procedure for cell procurement by apheresis.
       b) Risks and discomforts of the apheresis procurement procedure.
       c) Possibility of access device placement, along with its risks and discomforts, if peripheral venous access is unsuitable.
       d) Risks and side effects of growth factor and/or other pharmacologic agent(s), where applicable. **(cont'd)**

217

Table 5-1. General Requirements for Cellular Therapy Product Donors*† (Continued)

III. Determination of Donor Eligibility

A. All Donors

1) The facility shall define donor eligibility criteria to protect the safety of the intended recipient and, when applicable, to identify conditions that may adversely affect the potential therapeutic value of the cellular therapy product. For cord blood donors, in addition to evaluating the mother's medical history and infectious disease risk, the facility shall define criteria used to assess the infant donor for infection that may potentially affect the safety of the recipient or the therapeutic value of the cellular therapy product.

2) The facility shall evaluate donor eligibility according to these defined risk-based clinical and laboratory testing criteria.

3) Eligibility determination shall be performed and approved in a manner and timeframe that provides current relevant information and protects the safety of the intended recipient.

4) Donor eligibility records shall be reviewed before administration of a conditioning regimen to the recipient.

5) Procurement and use of products from allogeneic donors who do not meet eligibility criteria (determined to be incomplete or ineligible) shall require written approval by the facility's medical director and the recipient's physician.

6) For donors with incomplete screening or testing results, to complete eligibility determination, the facility shall:

   a) Complete eligibility determination if possible, or document in the records the reason that the eligibility could not be completed.

   b) Communicate results of the determination of donor eligibility to recipient's physician.

218

c) Provide a list of screening and testing that has been completed and a list of screening and testing that has not been completed.

d) Obtain urgent medical need documentation.

e) Label the product appropriately.

7) For donors who do not meet eligibility criteria, the facility shall keep records of:

a) Reason that the donor did not meet eligibility criteria.

b) Donor notification.

c) Identification and final disposition of previously collected products, if it is discovered that the donor does not meet eligibility criteria subsequent to procurement.

B. Specific Donor Requirements

1) Living Allogeneic Donors

a) Evaluation and approval of eligibility shall be performed before the recipient receives myeloablative marrow conditioning therapy or is otherwise prepared for donation. Interim health assessments, including psychosocial evaluation as appropriate, shall be performed by a qualified person or persons during the mobilization process (if applicable) and through procurement.

b) Donor eligibility records shall be reviewed before procurement-associated interventions (eg, drug or growth factor administration or line placement, biopsy, or surgical procedures).

c) If the donor is deemed ineligible before procurement, the procurement facility's medical director shall provide written approval.

(cont'd)

219

Table 5-1. General Requirements for Cellular Therapy Product Donors*† (Continued)

2) Autologous Donors

A health assessment specific to the donation procedure shall be performed by the autologous donor's physician before the scheduled procurement.

3) Mothers of Cord Blood Donors

a) Personal, family medical, and genetic histories of the family of the prospective cord blood donor shall be obtained before procurement but no later than 7 days after procurement.

b) If the medical history is obtained more than 7 days before procurement, the health history shall be reviewed for changes in infectious disease exposures in the birth mother.

c) In the case of a surrogate mother, her medical history shall be obtained and documented in addition to that of the biologic parents. A genetic history of the surrogate mother need not be obtained.

4) Cadaveric Donors

a) The evaluation of the donor's eligibility shall be performed by interviewing a family member or other relevant source.

b) When organs or tissues are procured from cadaveric donors, the facility shall specify the type of donor (DBD or DCD) by the protocol in use.

*Adapted with permission from Fontaine MJ, ed. Standards for cellular therapy product services. 6th ed. Bethesda, MD: AABB, 2013:70-3.
†Food and Drug Administration Guidance, August 8, 2007, "Eligibility Determination for Donors of Human Cells, Tissues, and Cellular and Tissue-Based Products (HCT/Ps)."

Table 5-2. Clinical Evaluation and Laboratory Testing of Donors*

	Living Allogeneic Donor	Autologous Donor[†]	Mother of Cord Blood Donor	Cadaveric Donor
I. Clinical Evaluation of Donor Suitability (to protect safety of the donor)				
General physical examination and health history	Yes	Yes	Yes	NA
Hemoglobinopathy risk[‡]	Yes	Yes	NA	NA
Anesthesia risk for marrow donors	Yes	Yes	NA	NA
Peripheral venous access for apheresis donors	Yes	Yes	No	No
Pregnancy in female donors	Yes	Yes	No	No
II. Clinical Evaluation of Donor Eligibility (to protect safety of the recipient)[§]				
Clinical and physical evidence of risk for, or symptoms of, transmissible disease[‖]	Yes	No	Yes	Yes
Immunization/vaccination history	Yes[¶]	No	Yes[¶]	Yes
Coroner and/or autopsy report (if available)	No	No	No	Yes

(cont'd)

221

Table 5-2. Clinical Evaluation and Laboratory Testing of Donors* (Continued)

	Living Allogeneic Donor	Autologous Donor[†]	Mother of Cord Blood Donor	Cadaveric Donor
History and behavioral risk for exposure to the following infectious agents or diseases:				
HIV	Yes	No	Yes	Yes
HBV	Yes	No	Yes	Yes
HCV	Yes	No	Yes	Yes
HTLV (viable, leukocyte-rich products only)	Yes	No	Yes	Yes
Syphilis	Yes	No	Yes	Yes
WNV	Yes	No	Yes	Yes
Vaccinia (smallpox vaccine)	Yes	No	Yes	Yes
Human TSEs	Yes	No	Yes	Yes
Malaria (travel or residence in malaria-endemic areas)	Yes	No	Yes	Yes
Rabies (contact with potentially rabid animal)	No	No	No	Yes
Chagas disease	Yes	No	Yes	Yes

III. Laboratory Testing#

HIV-1/2	Yes	Yes	Yes	Yes
HBV	Yes	Yes	Yes	Yes
HCV	Yes	Yes	Yes	Yes
Syphilis	Yes	Yes	Yes	Yes
HTLV-I/II (viable, leukocyte-rich products only)	Yes	Yes	Yes	Yes
CMV (viable, leukocyte-rich products only)	Yes	No	Yes	Yes**
HLA Type**	Yes††	No	N/A	Yes
ABO/Rh**	Yes	Yes	N/A	Yes
CBC (for apheresis and marrow donors)	Yes	Yes	N/A	N/A
WNV#	No	No	No	No
Trypanosoma cruzi (Chagas disease) #	No	No	No	No

(cont'd)

223

Table 5-2. Clinical Evaluation and Laboratory Testing of Donors* (Continued)

*Used with permission from Fontaine MJ, ed. Standards for cellular therapy product services. 6th ed. Bethesda, MD: AABB, 2013:74-6.

†Laboratory testing for infectious diseases is required only for autologous donors whose units will be cryopreserved.

‡Applies only to donors who will be mobilized.

§Relevant medical records as described in 21 CFR 1271.3(s).

||The relevant communicable diseases are described in 21 CFR 1271.3(r)(1)(i)(ii) and 1271.3(r)(2).

¶Evaluate for recent immunization and vaccination history.

#Perform tests for other relevant communicable diseases or disease agents as required by the FDA and interpret positive/reactive test results as described in 21 CFR 1271.80(d)(1).

**Testing shall be performed whenever this information is necessary for the selection and/or clinical use of a cellular therapy product.

††HLA-A, HLA-B, and HLA-DRB1 loci shall be determined. All typing used for the final selection of the donor shall use DNA-based technologies.

#West Nile virus is considered a relevant communicable agent or disease as defined under 21 CFR 1271.3(r)(2) by the FDA. However, at this time (2/2013), testing for WNV is not required. As of this date FDA has issued draft Guidance suggesting that T. cruzi will be considered a relevant communicable disease agent.

CBC = complete blood count; CMV = cytomegalovirus (anti-CMV, IgG and IgM); HBV = hepatitis B virus; HCV = hepatitis C virus; HIV = human immunodeficiency virus; HTLV = human T-cell lymphotropic virus; TSEs = transmissible spongiform encephalopathies; WNV = West Nile virus.

Table 5-3. Testing HCT/P Donors

Test	Blood	HCT/P	Reproductive Tissue	Source Plasma
ABO/Rh	X	X		
Antibody screen	X	X		
Hepatitis B surface antigen	X	X	X	X
Anti-HBc	X			X
Anti-HCV	X	X	X	X
Anti-HIV-1/2	X	X	X	X
Anti-HTLV- I/II	X	X	X	
Syphilis	X	X	X	X
HCV RNA	X	X		

(cont'd)

Table 5-3. Testing HCT/P Donors (Continued)

Test	Blood	HCT/P	Reproductive Tissue	Source Plasma
HIV-1 RNA	X	X		
WNV RNA	X			
Chlamydia trachomatis			X	
Neisseria gonorrhea			X	
T. cruzi	X			
Cytomegalovirus		X		
Sterility testing		X – cord blood, stem cells		

HBc = hepatitis B core antigen, HCV = hepatitis C virus, HIV-1/2 = human immunodeficiency virus types 1 and 2; HTLV-I/II = human T-lymphotropic virus types I and II; WNV = West Nile virus.

Table 5-4. Requirements for Labeling of Cellular Therapy Products*

(For labeling of regulated investigational products or licensed products, Standards 5.7.1.1 and 5.7.1.2 apply.)

Item No.	Element	Completion of Procurement†	In-Process Label†	Completion of Processing	Distribution and Issue‡
1	Unique alpha and/or numeric identifier of the product	P	P	P	P
2	Name of the product and modifiers§	P	P	P	P
3	Donor identifier or name‖	A		A¶	A¶
4	Date of procurement	R		R	R
5	Time of completion of procurement (time zone, if applicable)	R		R	R
6	Name of procurement facility/donor registry	R		R	R
7	Approximate product volume or weight (if applicable)	R		R	R

(cont'd)

227

Table 5-4. Requirements for Labeling of Cellular Therapy Products* (Continued)

Item No.	Element	Completion of Procurement†	In-Process Label†	Completion of Processing	Distribution and Issue‡
8	Names/volumes of anticoagulants and other additives (if applicable)	R		A¶	A¶
9	Recipient name and/or identifier (if known)	R	R	R	A¶
10	Expiration date and time (if applicable)			A#	A
11	ABO and Rh of the donor (if applicable)			R	R
12	Red cell compatibility (if applicable)				R
13	Recommended storage temperature (in degrees Celsius)	R		A	A
14	Name and address of the facility making the product available for distribution			R	R
15	Biohazard label (if applicable; see Reference Standard 5.7.1B)	A	A¶	A¶	A¶

#	Phrase				
16	Phrase: "Do Not Irradiate" (if applicable)		R	A"	A"
17	Phrase: "NOT EVALUATED FOR INFECTIOUS SUBSTANCES" and the statement "WARNING: Advise Patient of Communicable Disease Risks" (if applicable)	A	A"	A"	A"
18	Phrases: "Warning: Reactive Test Results for [name of disease agent or disease]" and "WARNING: Advise Patient of Communicable Disease Risks" (if applicable)	A	A"	A"	A"
19	Phrase: "Do Not Use Leukoreduction Filters" (if applicable)			A"	A"
20	Phrase: "For Autologous Use Only" (if applicable)	A	A"	A"	A"
21	Phrase: "For Use by Intended Recipient Only" (if applicable)		A"	A"	A"
22	Phrase: "Properly Identify Intended Recipient and Product"		A"	A"	A"

(cont'd)

Table 5-4. Requirements for Labeling of Cellular Therapy Products* (Continued)

Item No.	Element	Completion of Procurement†	In-Process Label†	Completion of Processing	Distribution and Issue‡
23	Phrase: "For Nonclinical Use Only" (if applicable)		A	A¶	A¶

*Used with permission from Fontaine MJ, ed. Standards for cellular therapy product services. 6th ed. Bethesda, MD: AABB, 2013:74-6.

†The in-process label may be used during processing and prior to distribution and issue.

‡The final labeling information for distribution shall be on or included with the container before the product is issued or transported.

§Includes content of container, including type of cellular therapy product, tissue, or organ, and anatomic orientation (eg, right or left).

ǁIn cases where donor anonymity must be preserved, such as with products from unrelated donor registries, this information is not required.

¶If affixing or attaching the applicable warnings and statements to the container is physically impossible, then the labeling must accompany the human cells, tissues, and cellular- and tissue-based products.

#If expiration date is not affixed to cryopreserved products at the end of processing, then records of stability studies shall be available to demonstrate expiration date at release of the cryopreserved product.

A = attached (may be permanently affixed); P = permanently affixed; R = accompanying records.

Table 5-5. Biohazard and Warning Labels on Cellular Therapy Products Collected, Processed, and/or Administered in the United States*

		Status				
		All Donor Screening and Testing Completed	Abnormal Results of Donor Screening	Abnormal Results of Donor Testing	Other Condition†	Urgent Medical Need
Donor Eligibility Determination Required [21 CFR 1271.45(b)]						
1	Allogeneic donors with incomplete donor eligibility determination‡	No	No	No		Yes
2	Allogeneic donors found ineligible					
	A first-degree or second-degree blood relative§	Yes	No/Yes	Yes		NA
	A first-degree or second-degree blood relative§	Yes	Yes	No		NA
	Unrelated donor‖	Yes	No/Yes	Yes		Yes
	Unrelated donor‖	Yes	Yes	No		Yes
	Unrelated donor	Yes	No	No	Yes	Yes

(cont'd)

231

Table 5-5. Biohazard and Warning Labels on Cellular Therapy Products Collected, Processed, and/or Administered in the United States* (Continued)

		Status				
	All Donor Screening and Testing Completed	Abnormal Results of Donor Screening	Abnormal Results of Donor Testing	Other Condition*	Urgent Medical Need	
Donor Eligibility Determination Not Required [21 CFR 1271.90(a)]						
3 Autologous donors¶						
Autologous donor#	No	No	No		NA	
Autologous donor**	Yes	No/Yes	Yes		NA	
Autologous donor**	Yes	Yes	No		NA	

Product Labels

	Biohazard Legend [per 21 CFR 1271.3(h)]	For Autologous Use Only	Not Evaluated for Infectious Substances	WARNING: Advise Patient of Communicable Disease Risks	WARNING: Reactive Test Results for (name of disease agent or disease)
Donor Eligibility Determination Required [21 CFR 1271.45(b)]					
1 Allogeneic donors with incomplete donor eligibility determination‡			X	X	
2 Allogeneic donors found ineligible					
A first-degree or second-degree blood relative§	X			X	X
A first-degree or second-degree blood relative§	X			X	

(cont'd)

233

Table 5-5. Biohazard and Warning Labels on Cellular Therapy Products Collected, Processed, and/or Administered in the United States* (Continued)

	Product Labels				
	Biohazard Legend [per 21 CFR 1271.3(h)]	For Autologous Use Only	Not Evaluated for Infectious Substances	WARNING: Advise Patient of Communicable Disease Risks	WARNING: Reactive Test Results for (name of disease agent or disease)
Unrelated donor||	X			X	X
Unrelated donor||	X			X	
Unrelated donor			X	X	
Donor Eligibility Determination Not Required [21 CFR 1271.90(a)]					
3 Autologous donors¶					
Autologous donor#		X	X		
Autologous donor**	X	X			X
Autologous donor**	X	X			

234

* Adapted with permission from AABB, America's Blood Centers, American Association of Tissue Banks, et al. Circular of information for the use of cellular therapy products. (November 2009) Bethesda, MD: AABB, 2009.

NOTE: Application of biohazard and warning labels extends outside the product described in 21 CFR 1271 based on adherence to professional standards and applies to unmanipulated HPC(M). Alternatively, unmanipulated HPC(M) is not regulated under 21 CFR 1271 but is included based on voluntary adherence to professional standards. Other cellular products which are not described in the 21 CFR 1271 [eg, HPC(A) from unrelated donors; HCP(CB)] are included in this table.

† Testing for infectious disease markers performed in non-CLIA-certified laboratory and/or using non-FDA cleared, approved, or licensed tests.

‡ The donor eligibility determination must be finalized during or after the use of the cellular therapy product. The results must be communicated to the treating physician [21 CFR 1271.60 (d)4]. Abnormal results of any screening or testing requires labeling as in item 2 in this table (21 CFR 1271.65 applies).

§ Notification of the recipient's and donor's physicians of abnormal screening and/or testing results is required. 21 CFR1271.65 (b)1.i.

|| 21 CFR 1271.65 (b)1.iii.

¶ Any abnormal donor screening or testing results (even though neither screening nor testing is mandated for this group of donors) require appropriate labeling [21 CFR 1271.90(b)]. 21 CFR 1271.90(a)(b).

21 CFR 1271.90(a)(1)(2).

** 21 CFR 1271.90(b)(1)(3).

CFR = Code of Federal Regulations; CLIA = Clinical Laboratory Improvement Amendments of 1988; FDA = Food and Drug Administration.

235

Table 5-6. Requirements for Labeling Shipping Containers*

Item No.	Element	Shipping Document[†]	Outer Shipping Container
1	Biohazard label (if applicable)	R	N/A
2	Phrase: "Do Not Irradiate" (if applicable)	R	A
3	Phrase: "Do Not X-Ray" (if applicable)	R	A
4	Phrases: "Medical Specimen" or "Human Cells for Transplantation" or equivalent	N/A	A
5	Date of distribution	R	A
6	Name and street address of receiving facility	R	A
7	Name and phone number of contact person at receiving facility	R	A
8	Name, street address, and phone number of the shipping facility	R	A

*Modified with permission from Fontaine MJ, ed. Standards for cellular therapy product services. 6th ed. Bethesda, MD: AABB, 2013:68.
[†]Shipping document shall be placed within the shipping container.
A = affixed or attached using a tie-tag; N/A = not applicable; R = accompanying records.

236

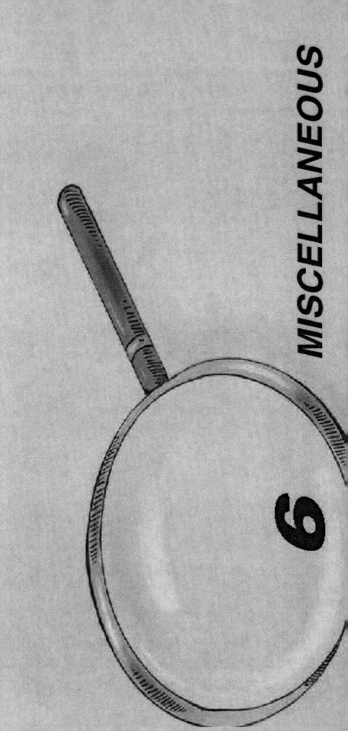

6

MISCELLANEOUS

Table 6-1. Metabolic Characteristics of Some Plasma Proteins*

Protein	Concentration (mg/mL)[†]	Molecular Weight (kDa)	Percentage Intravascular	FCR[‡] (%)	Change in FCR with ↓ Concentration	TER[§] (%)
IgG	12.1	150	45	6.7	→	3
IgA	2.6	$(160)_n$	42	25	constant	
IgM	0.9	950	76	18	constant	1-2
IgD	0.02	175	75	37	←	
IgE	0.0001	190	41	94	←	
Albumin	42±3.5	66	40	10	→	5-6
Fibrinogen	2-4	340	80	25	constant	2-3
C_3	1.5	240	53	56		
α_2-macro-globulin	2.6	820	100	8.2	constant	

*Used with permission from Chopek M, McCullough J. Protein and biochemical changes during plasma exchange. In: Berkman EM, Umlas J, eds. Therapeutic apheresis. Washington, DC: AABB, 1980:13-52.

[†]Concentration in normal serum or plasma.

[‡]Fractional catabolic rate (FCR): As percentage of intravascular mass per day.

[§]Transcapillary escape rate (TER): Total transfer of protein from intravascular to extravascular compartment as percentage of intravascular mass per hour.

238

Table 6-2. Pediatric Guidelines for Central Venous Catheter Size*

Patient Weight (in kg)	Catheter Size (Fr)†
<10	7
10-20	8
20-50	9
>50	9 or 11.5

*Adapted from Eder AF, Kim HC. Pediatric therapeutic apheresis. In: Herman JH, Manno CS, eds. Pediatric transfusion therapy. Bethesda, MD: AABB Press, 2002:471-508.
†For catheter manufactured by MedComp, Harleysville, Pennsylvania. Sizes may vary for other manufacturers' products.

Table 6-3. Common Needle Diameters*

Needle Gauge	External Diameter	
	Millimeters	Inches
16	1.651	0.0650
18	1.270	0.0500
20	0.902	0.0355
21	0.813	0.0320
22	0.711	0.0280
25	0.508	0.0200

*Used with permission from Brecher ME, Hay SN. Collected questions and answers. 9th ed. Bethesda, MD: AABB, 2008:112.

Table 6-4. Comparative Size and Weight of Blood Elements

Element	Diameter (in microns)	Density (specific gravity)
Red cell	7	1.093-1.096
Platelet	3	1.040
Plasma	—	1.025-1.029
Lymphocyte	10	1.070
Granulocyte	13	1.087-1.092

Table 6-5. Useful Diagnosis Codes for Therapeutic Apheresis*

Condition	ICD-10 Diagnosis Code(s)	ICD-9 Diagnosis Code(s)
ABO-incompatible hematopoietic stem cell transplantation—conditioning	Z76.82—awaiting transplant status	Use code for underlying disease prompting transplantation
ABO-incompatible hematopoietic stem cell transplantation—treatment for hemolysis or red cell aplasia	T80.30xA—initial encounter T80.30xD—subsequent encounter	996.85
ABO-incompatible solid organ transplantation—conditioning		Use code for underlying disease prompting transplantation
ABO-incompatible solid organ transplantation—treatment for hemolysis due to passenger lymphocyte syndrome	Kidney—T86.10 Liver—T86.40 Heart—T86.20 Lung—T86.819 Pancreas—T86.899 Intestine—T86.859	Kidney—996.81 Liver—996.82 Heart—996.83 Lung—996.84 Pancreas—996.86 Intestine—996.87
Acute disseminated encephalomyelitis (ADEM), noninfectious	G04.81	323.81
Acute disseminated encephalomyelitis (ADEM), postimmunization	G04.02	323.51

242

Acute disseminated encephalomyelitis (ADEM), postinfection	G04.01	136.9 and 323.61
Acute inflammatory demyelinating polyneuropathy (Guillain-Barré syndrome)	G61.0	357.0
Acute liver failure	K72.00	570
Age-related macular degeneration	H35.30	362.50
Amyloidosis, systemic (due to multiple myeloma)	E85.9 and C90.00	203.00
Amyotrophic lateral sclerosis	G12.21	335.20
ANCA (antineutrophil cytoplasmic antibodies)—rapidly progressive glomerulonephritis (crescentic glomerulonephritis)	N05.7	580.4
Antiglomerular basement membrane disease—pulmonary hemorrhage only	R04.89	786.30
Antiglomerular basement membrane disease—renal disease and pulmonary hemorrhage	M31.0	446.21
Antiglomerular basement membrane disease—renal disease only	M31.0	446.21

(cont'd)

243

Table 6-5. Useful Diagnosis Codes for Therapeutic Apheresis* (Continued)

Condition	ICD-10 Diagnosis Code(s)	ICD-9 Diagnosis Code(s)
Aplastic anemia; pure red cell aplasia	D60.9	284.81
Autoimmune hemolytic anemia—warm autoimmune hemolytic anemia; cold agglutinin disease	D59.1	283.0
Babesiosis	B60.0	088.82
Burn shock resuscitation	T79.4xxA—initial T79.4xxD—subsequent	958.4
Cardiac allograft rejection	T86.21	996.83
Catastrophic antiphospholipid syndrome	D68.61	289.81
Chronic focal encephalitis (Rasmussen encephalitis)	G04.81	323.81
Chronic inflammatory demyelinating polyradiculoneuropathy	G61.0	357.81
Coagulation factor inhibitors	D68.8	286.59
Cryoglobulinemia	D89.1	273.2
Cutaneous T-cell lymphoma—mycosis fungoides or Sezary syndrome	C82.60	202.20
Dermatomyositis	M33.90	710.3

Dilated cardiomyopathy	I42.0	425.4
Familial hypercholesterolemia	E78.0	272.0
Focal segmental glomerulosclerosis (either primary or recurrent)	N26.9	582.1
Graft-vs-host disease, acute	D89.810	279.51
Graft-vs-host disease, chronic	D89.811	279.52
Hemolytic uremic syndrome	D59.3	283.11
Henoch-Schonlein purpura	D69.0	287.0
Heparin-induced thrombocytopenia	D75.82	289.84
Hereditary hemochromatosis	E83.110	275.01
Hyperleukocytosis	D72.829	288.61
Hypertriglyceridemic pancreatitis	K85.9 and E78.1	577.0 and 272.1
Hyperviscosity in monoclonal gammopathies—multiple myeloma	C90.00	203.00
Hyperviscosity in monoclonal gammopathies—Waldenström macroglobulinemia	C88.0	273.3

(cont'd)

Table 6-5. Useful Diagnosis Codes for Therapeutic Apheresis* (Continued)

Condition	ICD-10 Diagnosis Code(s)	ICD-9 Diagnosis Code(s)
IgA nephropathy (Berger IgA nephropathy)	N02.8	583.9
Immune complex rapidly progressive glomerulonephritis	N01.9	580.4
Immune thrombocytopenia	D69.3	287.31
Inclusion body myositis	G72.41	359.71
Inflammatory bowel disease—Crohn disease	K50.90	555.9
Inflammatory bowel disease—ulcerative colitis	K51.90	556.9
Lambert-Eaton syndrome—associated with a malignancy	G73.1	199.1 and 358.31
Lambert-Eaton syndrome—no malignancy	G70.80	358.30
Lipoprotein(a) hyperlipoproteinemia	E78.5	272.4
Lung allograft rejection	T86.810	996.84
Malaria	B54	084.9
Multiple sclerosis	G35	340
Myasthenia gravis—acute exacerbation, in crisis	G70.01	358.01
Myasthenia gravis—prophylactic before surgery	G70.00	358.00

Myeloma cast nephropathy	C90.00	203.00
Nephrogenic systemic fibrosis	L90.5	701.8
Neuromyelitis optica (Devic syndrome)	G36.0	341.0
Overdose, venoms, and poisoning	Use code for specific agent	Use code for specific agent
Paraneoplastic neurologic syndromes—encephalitis or encephalomyelitis	G04.90	323.81
Paraneoplastic neurologic syndromes—cerebellar degeneration	G31.9 and D49.9	239.9 and 331.7
Paraneoplastic neurologic syndromes—peripheral neuropathy	G62.9 and D49.9	356.8
Paraneoplastic neurologic syndromes—polyneuropathy	D49.9 and G63	199.1 and 357.3
Paraneoplastic neurologic syndromes—other than those listed above	R76.8	Use code for symptom that triggered treatment and 795.79
Paraproteinemic polyneuropathies	G62.89	356.8
Pediatric autoimmune neuropsychiatric disorders associated with streptoccal infections (PANDAS)	M35.9 and Z86.19	279.49 and V12.09

(cont'd)

Table 6-5. Useful Diagnosis Codes for Therapeutic Apheresis* (Continued)

Condition	ICD-10 Diagnosis Code(s)	ICD-9 Diagnosis Code(s)
Pemphigus vulgaris	L10.0	694.4
Peripheral vascular disease	I73.9	443.9
Phytanic acid storage disease (Refsum disease)	G60.1	356.3
POEMS (polyneuropathy, organomegaly, endocrinopathy, M protein, and skin changes)	E88.89	273.8
Polycythemia vera and erythrocytosis	D45 and D75.1	238.4
Polymyositis	M33.20	710.4
Posttransfusion purpura	D69.51	287.41
Psoriasis—any type except arthropathic	L40.9	696.1
Psoriasis—arthropathic	L40.50	696.0
Red cell alloimmunization in pregnancy	036.091—first trimester 036.092—second trimester 036.093—third trimester	656.13
Renal transplantation—antibody-mediated rejection	T86.11	996.81

Renal transplantation—conditioning for crossmatch or ABO-incompatible transplant or for focal segmental glomerulosclerosis	T86.19	Use code for underlying disease prompting transplantation
Rheumatoid arthritis—refractory	M06.9	714.0
Schizophrenia	F20.9	295.90
Scleroderma (progressive systemic sclerosis)	M34.9	710.1
Sepsis with multiorgan failure	A41.9 and R65.11	Use code for organism causing sepsis and 995.92
Sickle cell anemia—acute chest syndrome	D57.01	282.62 and 517.3
Sickle cell anemia—acute stroke	D57.1 and I63.8	282.62 and 434.91
Sickle cell anemia—acute stroke prophylaxis	D57.1 and Z79.899	282.60
Sickle cell anemia—hepatic sequestration	D57.1 and K76.89	282.69 and 573.8
Sickle cell anemia—intrahepatic cholestasis	D57.1 and K71.0	282.69 and 576.8
Sickle cell anemia—multiorgan failure	D57.01 and R65.11	995.94 and code for specific organ failing

(cont'd)

Table 6-5. Useful Diagnosis Codes for Therapeutic Apheresis* (Continued)

Condition	ICD-10 Diagnosis Code(s)	ICD-9 Diagnosis Code(s)
Sickle cell anemia—pregnancy	O99.011—first trimester O99.012—second trimester O99.013—third trimester	648.2X and 282.60
Sickle cell anemia—priapism	D57.1 and N48.32	282.62 and 607.3
Sickle cell anemia—prophylaxis before surgery	D57.1 and Z79.899	282.60 and code for reason for surgery
Sickle cell anemia—splenic sequestration	D57.02	282.69 and 289.52
Sickle cell anemia—vaso-occlusive pain crisis	D57.00	282.69 and 443.89
Stiff-person syndrome	G25.82	333.91
Sudden sensorineural hearing loss	H90.5	388.2
Sydenham chorea	I02.9	392.9
Systemic lupus erythematosus	M32.9	710.0
Thrombocytosis (primary or secondary)	D47.3	238.71
Thrombotic microangiopathy—drug associated	M31.1	446.6

Thrombotic microangiopathy—hematopoietic stem cell transplant associated	T86.03	446.6
Thrombotic thrombocytopenic purpura	M31.1	446.6
Thyroid storm	E05.90	242.91
Toxic epidermal necrolysis	L51.2	695.15
Voltage-gated potassium channel antibody disease	D89.9	279.8
Wegener granulomatosis (necrotizing respiratory granulomatosis)	A50.02 or M31.30	446.4
Wilson disease, fulminant	E83.01	275.1

*Adapted with permission from Winters JL, King K, eds. Therapeutic apheresis: A physician's handbook. 4th ed. Bethesda, MD: AABB, 2013.